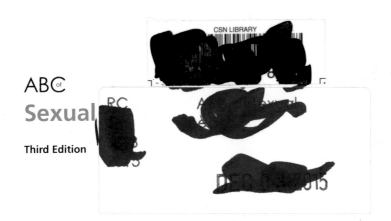

ABC of
Sexual
Third Edition

DATE DUE

Brodart Co.   Cat. # 55 137 001   Printed in USA

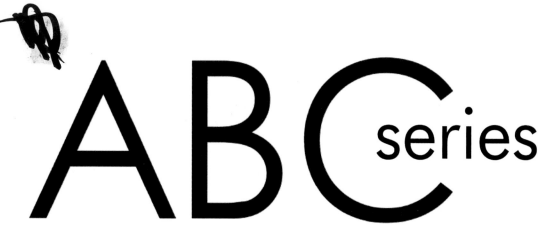

ABC series

An outstanding collection of resources for everyone in primary care

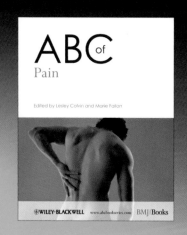

ABC of Pain

Edited by Lesley Colvin and Marie Fallon

WILEY-BLACKWELL www.abcbookseries.com BMJ|Books

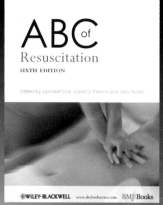

ABC of Resuscitation

SIXTH EDITION

Edited by Jasmeet Soar, Gavin D. Perkins and Jerry Nolan

WILEY-BLACKWELL www.abcbookseries.com BMJ|Books

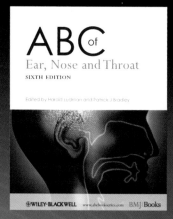

ABC of Ear, Nose and Throat

SIXTH EDITION

Edited by Harold Ludman and Patrick J Bradley

WILEY-BLACKWELL www.abcbookseries.com BMJ|Books

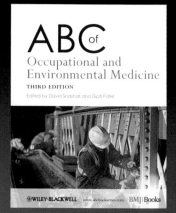

ABC of Occupational and Environmental Medicine

THIRD EDITION

Edited by David Snashall and Dipti Patel

WILEY-BLACKWELL www.abcbookseries.com BMJ|Books

The *ABC* series contains a wealth of indispensable resources for GPs, GP registrars, junior doctors, doctors in training and all those in primary care

► **Highly illustrated, informative and a practical source of knowledge**

► **An easy-to-use resource, covering the symptoms, investigations, treatment and management of conditions presenting in day-to-day practice and patient support**

► **Full colour photographs and illustrations aid diagnosis and patient understanding of a condition**

For more information on all books in the *ABC* series, including links to further information, references and links to the latest official guidelines, please visit:

www.abcbookseries.com

WILEY-BLACKWELL

BMJ|Books

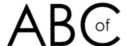

Sexual Health

Third Edition

EDITED BY

Kevan Wylie MD FRCP FRCPsych FRCOG FECSM

Consultant in Sexual Medicine, Sheffield, UK;
Honorary Professor of Sexual Medicine, University of Sheffield;
President, World Association for Sexual Health

WILEY Blackwell

BMJ|Books

BMJ Books is an imprint of BMJ Publishing Group Limited, used under licence by John Wiley & Sons.

Registered office: John Wiley & Sons, Ltd, The Atrium, Southern Gate, Chichester, West Sussex, PO19 8SQ, UK

Editorial offices: 9600 Garsington Road, Oxford, OX4 2DQ, UK

The Atrium, Southern Gate, Chichester, West Sussex, PO19 8SQ, UK

111 River Street, Hoboken, NJ 07030-5774, USA

For details of our global editorial offices, for customer services and for information about how to apply for permission to reuse the copyright material in this book please see our website at www.wiley.com/wiley-blackwell

Library of Congress Cataloging-in-Publication Data

ABC of sexual health / edited by Kevan Wylie. – Third edition.

  p. ; cm. – (ABC series)

  Preceded by ABC of sexual health / edited by John M. Tomlinson. 2nd edition. 2005.

  Includes bibliographical references and index.

  ISBN 978-1-118-66569-5 (pbk.)

  I. Wylie, Kevan, editor. II. Series: ABC series (Malden, Mass.)

  [DNLM: 1.   Sexual Dysfunction, Physiological. 2.   Sexual Behavior.   WP 610]

  RC556

  616.6′9–dc23

                                    2014049377

A catalogue record for this book is available from the British Library.

Wiley also publishes its books in a variety of electronic formats. Some content that appears in print may not be available in electronic books.

Cover image: mating-ladybugs-6163495 © isgaby/iStockphoto

Typeset in 9.25/12 MinionPro by Laserwords Private Ltd, Chennai, India

Printed and bound in Malaysia by Vivar Printing Sdn Bhd

1   2015

Contents

Series Foreword

Why do we need an *ABC of Sexual Health*? The answer is straightforward; the subject is important, which is often not advised about and often not taught in medical school or at the post graduate level. When questioned as to what is important in a happy marriage, sexual relationships were considered very important and when patients had concerns they wanted more information and healthcare professionals to **initiate** discussion. Far too often healthcare professionals wait for the patient to raise the subject, whereas they need to be more proactive. In a recent survey, of more than 450 cardiologists, 70% gave no advice, 54% saying there was a lack of patient initiative and 43% saying they didn't have the time. In this vacuum, *ABC of Sexual Health* is clearly needed so that healthcare professionals can know more about this unmet need.

In 1970, the World Health Organization summarised the right to sexual health, including it as part of the fundamental rights of an individual.

- A capacity to enjoy and control sexual health and reproductive behaviour in accordance with social and personal ethics
- Freedom from fear, shame, guilt, false beliefs and other factors inhibiting sexual response and impairing sexual relationships
- Freedom from organic disorders, diseases and deficiencies that interfere with sexual and reproductive function

So nearly 50 years later it is right that we ask ourselves "how are we doing?" The short answer is: not well enough. There are many disciplines involved and access to these should become routine, and this book forms an essential beginning.

Dr. Graham Jackson
Cardiologist and Chairman
of the Sexual Advice Association

Contributors

Richard Balon

Departments of Psychiatry and Behavioral Neurosciences and AnesthesiologyWayne State University School of Medicine, Detroit, MI, USA

Yitzchak M. Binik

Department of Psychology, Alan Edwards Centre for Research on PainMcGill University, Montréal, QC, Canada

Johannes Bitzer

Department of Obstetrics and Gynecology, University Hospital Basel, Basel Switzerland

Lori A. Brotto

Department of Obstetrics and Gynaecology, University of British Columbia, Vancouver, Canada

Chris Bunker

Department of Dermatology, University College Hospital, London, London, UK

Department of Dermatology, Chelsea and Westminster Hospital, London, UK

Eli Coleman

Program in Human Sexuality, University of Minnesota, Minneapolis, MN, USA

Brian Daines

Department of Psychiatry, University of Sheffield, Sheffield, UK

Dominic Davies

Pink Therapy, London, UK

Seth Davis

Faculty of Medicine, University of Toronto, Toronto, ON, Canada

John Dean

Clinical Director, Gender & Sexual Medicine, Devon Partnership NHS Trust, Exeter, UK

Melissa A. Farmer

University of Toronto, Toronto, ON, Canada

Alan Edwards Centre for Research on Pain, McGill University, Montreal, QC, Canada

Julie A. Fitter

Porterbrook Clinic, Sheffield Health and Social Care NHS Foundation Trust, Sheffield, UK

Lin Fraser

Psychotherapist, San Francisco, CA, USA

Woet L. Gianotten

Erasmus University Medical Centre, Rotterdam, The Netherlands, University Medical Centre, Utrecht, The Netherlands

David Goldmeier

Sexual Medicine, St Marys Hospital, London, UK

Honorary Senior Lecturer, Imperial College London, St Marys Hospital, London, UK

Irwin Goldstein

Sexual Medicine, Alvarado Hospital, San Diego CA, USA

Don Grubin

Institute of Neuroscience, Newcastle University, Newcastle upon Tyne, UK

Honorary Consultant Forensic Psychiatrist, Northumberland Tyne and Wear NHS Foundation Trust, Newcastle upon Tyne, UK

Geoffrey Hackett

Good Hope Hospital, Sutton Coldfield, Birmingham, UK

Trudy Hannington

Leger Clinic, Doncaster, UK

The College of Sexual and Relationship Therapists (COSRT), Doncaster, London, UK

T. Hugh Jones

Robert Hague Centre for Diabetes and Endocrinology, Barnsley Hospital NHS Foundation Trust, Barnsley, UK

Department of Human Metabolism, School of Medicine and Biomedical Sciences, University of Sheffield, Sheffield, UK

Gail A. Knudson

University of British Columbia, Vancouver, BC, Canada

Ellen T. M. Laan

Department of Sexology and Psychosomatic Obstetrics and Gynaecology, Academic Medical Centre, University of Amsterdam, Amsterdam, The Netherlands

Roy J. Levin

Sexual Physiology Laboratory, Porterbrook Clinic, Sheffield, UK

Fraukje E. F. Mevissen

Work and Social Psychology Department, Maastricht University, Maastricht, The Netherlands

Ruth Murphy

Consultant Dermatologist, Nottingham University Teaching Hospitals, Nottingham, UK

Sara Nasserzadeh

Psychosexual Therapist, Connections ABC, New York, NY, USA

Sue Newsome

Sex Therapist & Tantra Teacher, London, UK.

Sharon J. Parish

Department of Psychiatry, Weill Cornell Medical College, New York, USA

New York Presbyterian Hospital/ Westchester Division, White Plains, New York, USA

Yacov Reisman

Men's Health Clinics, Department of Urology Amstell and Hospital Amstelveen and Bovenij Hospital Amsterdam, The Netherlands

Ross Runciman

Wotton Lawn Hospital, Horton Road, Gloucester, UK

Manu Shah

Burnley General Hospital, East Lancashire, UK

Francesca Tripodi

Institute of Clinical Sexology, Rome, Italy

Jacques van Lankveld

Open University, Heerlen, The Netherlands

Marcel D. Waldinger

Division of Pharmacology, Utrecht Institute for Pharmaceutical Sciences, Utrecht University, Utrecht, The Netherlands

Alison K. Wood

Old Age Psychiatry, Sheffield, UK

Kevan Wylie

Sexual Medicine, Porterbrook Clinic and Urology, Sheffield, UK

Honorary Professor of Sexual Medicine, University of Sheffield, UK

President, World Association for Sexual Health, Minneapolis, USA

CHAPTER 1

Psychosexual Development

Brian Daines

University of Sheffield, Sheffield, UK

OVERVIEW

- Psychosexual development is not limited to childhood and adolescence but extends through adult life
- Early psychoanalytic views of the process are still influential but more recent ideas such as consumerist and feminist perspectives offer a more societal emphasis
- It is important to consider the impact of the aspects of law and culture that relate to psychosexual development
- Clinicians need to be aware of the implications of these issues and the various factors impacting on development in their consultations with patients.

Introduction

Interest in psychosexual development has tended to focus around managing problems, particularly those associated with risks and their management. These areas include sexual abuse in childhood and early adolescence, unwanted pregnancy and sexually transmitted diseases (STDs) in adolescence and early adulthood and functional sexual difficulties in adults. In contrast, the interest, for example of adolescents has been shown to be more in the rite of passage and recreational aspects of sexual activity. There has also been a concentration on childhood and adolescence, with adult psychosexual development being a poor relation and any emphasis for older people being on dysfunctions and disorders rather than the expected course of development. Development through the life cycle involves important areas such as sexual identity, couple relationship issues, fertility and ageing.

Psychoanalytic views

Probably, the most familiar schema of sexual development in childhood and adolescence is that proposed by Freud (Table 1.1). This still has currency in many modern textbooks despite having long been superseded, not only outside of the world of psychoanalysis, but also generally among psychotherapists. A primary criticism is that it pathologizes variations in sexual development, in particular

Table 1.1 Freud on psychosexual development

Oral stage 0–2 years
Desires are focussed on the lips and mouth. The mother becomes the first love-object, a displacement from the earliest object of desire, the breast

Anal stage 2–4 years of age
In this stage, the anus is the new auto-erotic object with pleasure being obtained from controlling bladder and bowel movement

Phallic stage 4–7 years of age
In this third stage, awareness of and touching the genitals is the primary source of pleasure

Latency period 7–12 years of age
During this time, sexual development is more or less suspended and sexual urges are repressed

Genital phase 13 years + (or from puberty on)
In this final phase, sexual urges are direct onto opposite sex peers with the primary focus of pleasure of the genitals

gay and lesbian relationships. With the passage of time, Freud's emphasis on instinct and drive was replaced by highlighting the importance of relating and relationship and then broadened to recognize the importance of learning and culture. Freud's theories assume that children are caught in hidden conflicts between their fears and their desires, whereas the environmental learning view is of identification through observation and imitation. Modern psychoanalytic views include a wide range of innovative ideas such as that the various dynamics in childhood produce a psychosexual core which is unstable, elusive and never felt to be really owned.

Consumerist view

At the other end of the spectrum are ideas that take a societal perspective, such as consumer culture bringing sexuality into the world of commerce. Sex is used to sell products through sexiness and physical attractiveness being closely connected with the goods we buy and are seen to own. This aspect of sex and consumerism is particularly directed towards girls and women. A further development is when sex itself is marketed as pleasure or the idea of sexual self-expression is promoted. The world is sexualized, and there is a seduction into the world of responding to sexual impulse. On the Internet in particular, representations of the body become products to buy. This becomes the world into which children and adolescents are socialized and encouraged to participate. As we grow up, sexuality becomes increasingly focussed on technique

---

ABC of Sexual Health, Third Edition. Edited by Kevan Wylie.

and performance with a tendency for it to come to resemble work risking the loss of much of its intimate and caring qualities.

Feminist views

The feminist perspective is that gender shapes our personality and social life and that our sexual desires, feelings and preferences are deeply rooted by our gender status. The identification between mothers and daughters leads girls to become very relationship-orientated. This promotes the connection of sex with intimacy and the valuing of its caring and sharing aspects. It develops as a means of communication and intimacy rather than a source of erotic pleasure. In contrast, boys develop a more detached relationship with their mothers and do not have the same kind of identification with their fathers and this leads them to be more goal-orientated around sexuality. There is more of an emphasis on pleasure and on performance. It is also argued that girls' identification with their mothers makes their heterosexual identification weaker than that of boys.

Definition of childhood and adolescence

The nature of childhood and adolescence has been subject to debate and controversy. Whilst all acknowledge that the nature of both has changed in Western culture over the centuries, there is some dispute about when the idea of childhood as a distinctive phase began, and it has been suggested that the idea we have currently of adolescence did not exist before the beginning of the twentieth century. It has also been argued that the concept of childhood makes children more vulnerable including to sexual exploitation and abuse. The idealization of childhood may also contribute to the sexual attraction of children to certain adults.

The impact of law and culture

Aspects of the definitions of childhood and adolescent become enshrined in law particularly in defining the age of consent for sex and what kinds of sexual practices are legal. It also defines a framework for marriage, and alongside this are cultural issues about the acceptability of sexual relationships outside of this. In different countries, the age of consent varies from 12 to 21 for heterosexual, gay and lesbian relationships, but in many countries same-sex relationships are still illegal. The position is complicated by the fact that these arrangements are often subject to review and potential change.

Although it is clearly interwoven, law is only one of the forces at work here as family, religion, culture and mass media also influence teenage attitudes and behaviour. All these forces work together in ways that overlap, support and sometimes contradict one another in the emergence of a normative version of teenage sexuality.

Childhood development

Young children show behaviours that indicate awareness of sexual organs and pleasuring very early and preschoolers are often puzzled by sexual anatomical differences. By the age of 2 or 3, they become aware of their gender and aspects of gender role. Children often have a need for the validation and correction of their sexual learning, but adults often do not feel well-informed about childhood sexuality and, as a consequence, are not confident about how to respond in their care of children. Play such as doctors and nurses and looking at genitals are all common during the preschool and early school years and as many as half of all adults remember this kind of childhood sexual play. The discovery of such activities can give parents and caregivers an opportunity to educate and share values. An example of this would be that another person should not touch them in a way that makes them feel afraid, confused or uncomfortable. Activities between children such as those involving pain, simulated or real penetration or oral–genital contact should raise concerns and may be related to exposure to inappropriate adult entertainment or indicate sexual abuse. School-age children are usually able to understand basic information about sexuality and sexual development and may look to various sources for information, such as friends and the Internet.

Adolescent development

Early teenage development can be characterized by concerns about normality, appearance and attractiveness. As girls' physical development is usually more advanced than that of boys of the same age, they may experience sexual feelings earlier and be attracted to older, more physically mature boys. Those who have early intercourse have been found to have lower self-esteem than virgins, unlike boys for whom intercourse is more socially acceptable. For boys, there is evidence that both peers and families can potentially either support or undermine sexual development and that health care providers may have more influence than they presume. The middle phase sees the exploration of gender roles and an awareness of sexual orientation. Fantasies are idealistic and romanticized, and sexual experimentation and activity often begin in relationships that are often brief and self-serving. Online communication is used for relationship formation and sexual self-exploration but also carries risks of unwanted or inappropriate sexual solicitation.

In late adolescence, there is an acceptance of sexual identity and intimate relationships are based more on giving and sharing, rather than the earlier exploration and romanticism. Research among students has suggested that first experiences of intercourse in late adolescence lead males to be more satisfied with their appearance, whereas females became slightly less satisfied. In all this, it is important to bear in mind the wide variability in individual adolescent development which is evident to all who work with this age group.

Factors impacting on development

Impairment or delay in psychosexual development can be caused by a number of factors including:

- physical developmental disorders
- some chronic illnesses and treatments
- lack of appropriate educational opportunities
- absent or poor role models

Promoters of early sexualization include

- inappropriate comments and attention from adults
- sexual abuse
- viewing pornography
- sexual experiences with peers at a young age

The effects of early puberty in girls can include early sexual behaviour and an increased number of lifetime sexual partners. Research has confirmed that both early puberty and late puberty in girls are associated with low self-esteem. Disruption in development can also be brought about by:

- education into misleading or inaccurate information about sex
- experiencing or witnessing sexually abusive or violent acts
- sexual humiliations or rejections

Adult development

The main developmental tasks for young adults are completing the development of adequate sexual confidence and functioning and establishing the potential for desired couple relationships. The latter may range through a spectrum of possible arrangements from

Table 1.2 Adult psychosexual development tasks

Consolidating sexual identity and orientation (teens and twenties)

Developing adequate sexual confidence and functioning (late teens and twenties)

Establishing the potential for desired couple relationships (late teens and twenties)

Managing issues around fertility (twenties, thirties and forties)

Adjusting to the effects of ageing (forties onwards)

Facing and dealing with loss (forties or fifties onwards)

Adjusting to illness and disability (at any point but particularly in the elderly)

Table 1.3 Learning points for clinicians

Expressions of sexuality in childhood need to be carefully assessed to avoid missing situations that need intervention or pathologizing expression that fall within the range of normal development

Developmental issues and adolescent needs should not to be obscured by preoccupations about risk

Care needs to be taken that valid developments in sexual orientation and preferences are not pathologized

There needs to be an awareness of the relevance of developmental issues throughout the life cycle

Problems related to sexuality may be partly a result of a difficulty in transition through a developmental stage or of a past stage that was not successfully negotiated

It is important to be aware of the assumptions and values that underlay ideas about normal development and the potential conflict between societal concerns and individual aspirations

marriage to one-night stands as lifestyle choices. Over the period of fertility, decisions about children are taken either as choices or responses to physical limitations. This is followed by more marked accommodation in response to ageing. The decrease in frequency of sexual activity at this point is thought to involve relational as well as physical factors. Social attitudes tend to claim sex as the province of the young and fit and that there is something distasteful about interest in sex and sexual activity beyond young adulthood, particularly in the elderly. Later in life, but potentially at any point, adjustments to illness or disability may have to be made (Table 1.2 and 1.3).

Further reading

Bancroft, J. (2009) *Human Sexuality and its Problems*, 3rd edn. Churchill Livingstone, Edinburgh ch.

Hornberger, L.L. (2006) Adolescent psychosocial growth and development. *Journal of Pediatric and Adolescent Gynecology*, **19**, 243–246.

Seidman, S. (2003) *The Social Construction of Sexuality*. Norton, New York.

CHAPTER 2

Physical Aspects of Sexual Development

Woet L. Gianotten[1,2]

[1]Erasmus University Medical Centre, Rotterdam, The Netherlands
[2]University Medical Centre, Utrecht, The Netherlands

OVERVIEW

- This chapter focuses on the nature aspects of female–male development and differences
- Step 1 takes place at the conception when the genotypic sex is determined by XX or XY
- Step 2 starts 7 weeks later with the development of the gonadal sex. Without interference of testosterone, the default is female. With testosterone, the gonads, the genitals and the brain will 'grow male'
- From birth to puberty, there is no activity of gonadal hormones
- Puberty is the last phase of differentiation and preparation for adult life and reproduction
- After puberty, the gonadal hormones have only activational function and no more organizational function.

Introduction

Talking about sexuality is also talking about female/male differences, a major topic in the history of our human race. Depending on time and culture more or less value has been attributed to the biological, the psychological or the social influences, sometimes denying the importance of specific elements. A striking example of that nurture–nature debate happened three decades ago in Western culture. Then, the predominant idea was that education (=nurture) was the major reason for the difference between the sexes, and the biological influence was nearly completely denied. So, the toys for children were adjusted. Girls were given Dinky Toys and boys got dolls. But nature proved stronger than education. The dolls were used as the enemy and the Dinky Toys were sometimes pampered by the girls. One cannot simply erase millions of years of evolution.

Talking female–male differences is very tricky, as it easily can be seen as discriminating one group. However, one cannot educate well without understanding the differences. Two important aspects of wisdom are needed to properly deal with that: *Judgement* and *relative value*. Judgement: male is not better than female, female not better than male. Relative value: Take the size of people. Men tend to be taller than women. But some women are taller than some men. So, it

is not in 100% true. Or take sexual desire (for which testosterone is the major fuel). The man, having a much higher level of testosterone, will have more sexual desire than his female partner. But that stands not 100% of the time, and not in 100% of the couples.

The very first moment of difference takes place at conception when the genotypic sex is settled. The karyotype (with chromosomal constitution XX or XY) harbours the genetic information for the next step. There is no sexual dimorphism in the first 6 weeks of development or in the primordial gonads. The next important step is the development of gonadal sex. The default is female. Without interfering, the gonads, the genitals and the brain will 'grow female'. However, in the presence of the Y chromosome, the primordial gonads will develop into testes and then emit hormones that will steer the genitals and the brain in the male direction. When orchestrating this development of the genitals and the brain, the sex hormones have an organizational function, whereas in later life, after the development is complete, they have an activational function, guiding sexual and reproductive behaviour. The hormonal influence results in the phenotypic sex, defined by the primary and secondary sexual characteristics of that individual. Hormones play also an important role in the formation of a person's gender identity, but they are only part of the total picture as many rearing and environmental factors add spice to that development.

Next to the mainstream, there are many sideways in this process of sexual differentiation with changes in genotypic sex, gonadal sex, phenotypic sex and/or gender identity. Inconsistencies in the biological indicators of sex, traditionally known as intersex or intersex disorders, are nowadays called 'disorders of sex development (DSD)'. Inconsistencies in gender identity without involvement of the genital tract usually are called 'Gender Identity Disorder (GID)'. See Chapter 26 (gender dysphoria section).

In this chapter, we deal only with the mainstream development, starting with intrauterine development, then the period between birth and puberty and then puberty.

Intrauterine development

The four relevant anatomical structures for sexuality development are the gonads, the Wolffian system, the Müllerian system and the brain. In the first 6 weeks after conception, male and female developments are the same. Becoming female is in a way the 'default process'. Without the Y chromosome, the development will

ABC of Sexual Health, Third Edition. Edited by Kevan Wylie.
© 2015 John Wiley & Sons, Ltd. Published 2015 by John Wiley & Sons, Ltd.

continue towards female. Then the primordial gonads will develop into female gonads (ovaries), with atrophy of the Wolffian system and development of the Müllerian system into female internal genitalia. Intrauterine female development is independent of ovarian hormones!

The default system of becoming female happens also in the brain. The foetal brain grows very fast and especially in the period between 6 and 18 weeks of pregnancy, the layout for many important and permanent structures is settled. The 'undisturbed' (i.e. without testicular hormones) wiring in the brain 'grows female', giving a strong base for the later typical female behaviour. This process is not the result of oestrogens. Although oestrogens are abundantly present in both female and male foetuses, they are so strongly bound to alpha-foetoproteins that they cannot enter the foetal brain compartment.

What about male development? With chromosomal pattern XY, a gene on the Y chromosome (SRY or Sex determining Region of the Y chromosome) causes a complex cascade of steps, bending this process towards male development. This SRY contains the code for the production of a testis-determining protein, which in turn causes the primitive gonads to become testes.

Then, three very relevant processes deserve to be mentioned, all beginning at around 6 weeks after conception:

1 The Leydig cells of the testes start producing hormones. Testosterone (T) is responsible for stimulation of the Wolffian system to develop into male internal genitalia. Later in the foetal life, Dihydrotestosterone (DHT) is responsible for development of the male external genitalia, and INSL3 for the testicular descent.
2 The Sertoli cells of the testes start producing MIS (Müllerian Inhibiting Substance, also called AMH or anti-Müllerian Hormone), by which the Müllerian tubes are suppressed and disappear, preventing the development of female genitalia.
3 The foetal brain becomes bathed in these two hormones T and MIS, by which the wiring in the brain 'grows male'.

This supposed 'dimorphic wiring' can be seen at a macroscopic level in some brain areas. At 26 weeks of pregnancy, the corpus callosum (connecting the left and the right side of the brain) is bigger in the female foetus. The sexual dimorphic nucleus of the preoptic area (SDN-POA) of the amygdala (responsible for sexual behaviour) is in the human male twice as big as in the female.

As the construction of human beings is not like in a factory assembly line, there is much variety in intrauterine development. We know for instance about the variety in intrauterine exposure to testosterone. This shows in later life in the 2D/4D ratio (the difference between the length of the second and that of the fourth finger). A higher 2D/4D ratio is an expression of lower intrauterine T-exposition. So, females have a higher 2D/4D ratio than males. Women with higher 2D/4D ratios have more verbal skills, whereas women with lower ratios have a better sense of spatial direction. On such basis, many relations are found with toy preference, personality characteristics, sexual orientation and cognitive profile (spatial, verbal and mathematical abilities). Males generally outperform females on math and spatial tasks, whereas women outperform males on verbal fluency and fine motor skills.

As mentioned earlier, talking sex differences is a sensitive topic. In stark contrast to the differences model stands the gender similarities hypothesis. This states that males and females are alike on most – but not all – psychological variables. With her meta-analyses of research on gender differences, Janet Hyde supported this gender similarities hypothesis with as few notable exceptions some motor behaviours and some aspects of sexuality, which show large gender differences and aggression showing a gender difference moderate in magnitude. What is the reason behind those differences? They are the result of thousands of generations of evolution. All geared to preservation of the species. After all that is what we have to do and what nature dictates us. This chapter concludes with a small hint in that direction. Several times a day, the male foetus has erections (from 26 weeks of pregnancy), preparing him for his evolutionary task of reproduction. Although not yet shown in ultrasound examination, the female foetus most probably will have the corresponding perivaginal hypercirculation, preparing her as well for her reproductive future.

From birth to puberty

Immediately after birth, the hormonal levels of the newborn baby drop considerably. Then, the male baby goes through another androgen surge, probably for further masculinization of his central nervous system. This surge takes several months, whereas female androgen levels stay very low. From the age of 6 months, both boys and girls have very low levels of sex steroids (see Figures 2.1 and 2.2). That is maybe surprising, as already in these early years girls and boys differ in many areas: play, socializing, competition, fine motor skills, verbal fluency and so on. See Brizendine. Very probably, those differences are the result of the dimorphic wiring in the central nervous system.

The next endocrine activity comes from the adrenal glands. The 'adrenarche' can start from age 6 in girls and age 8 in boys with an increase in the production of androgens. This probably explains the

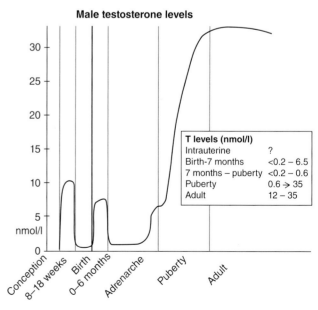

Figure 2.1 Male testosterone levels

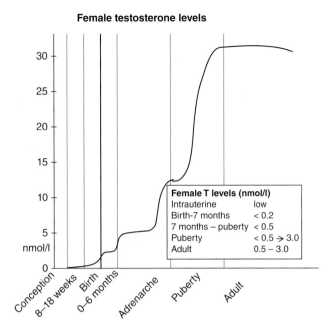

Female testosterone levels

Female T levels (nmol/l)	
Intrauterine	low
Birth-7 months	< 0.2
7 months – puberty	< 0.5
Puberty	< 0.5 → 3.0
Adult	0.5 – 3.0

Figure 2.2 Female testosterone levels

early growth of axillary and pubic hair and maybe the early masturbation in part of the girls.

Puberty

During puberty, body and mind undergo many changes in the direction of independence from parents, and towards sexual partnership and reproduction. The adult secondary sexual characteristics and reproductive capacity develop and the growth spurt takes place, accompanied by many changes in sexual thoughts and behaviour, in the relation to the opposite sex and in the relation to the surrounding society.

All these processes are orchestrated by the hypothalamic–pituitary–gonadal axis, but they are also influenced by genetic and environmental signals. The hypothalamus secretes (in pulses) GnRH and the first endocrine change in puberty is a nocturnal increase in the luteinising hormone (LH) pulse, developing in a day/night rhythm.

Boys start puberty with testicular growth, approximately half a year later than the initiation of breast development in girls (which is already preceded by the female increase in height velocity).

For clinical comparison, a five-stage classification system for boys and for girls was developed by Tanner.

Boy–man

In boys, the increase in nocturnal LH-pulses goes with an increase in testosterone. Many a mother recognizes the start of her son's puberty by the disappearance of the puppy smell, due to small amounts of androstenedione in his sweat. The clinical sign of puberty's onset is a testicular length greater than 2.5 cm or a volume greater than 4 ml. Usually, the right testis grows larger and the left testis hangs lower in the scrotum. Testosterone causes also the growth of pubic hair, elongation of the penis, lengthening of the vocal cords and changes in the larynx and cricothyroid cartilage. Facial hair starts growing and the skin reacts with acne. The first sign of spermatogenesis (at age 11–15) is the detection of sperm in early-morning urine. Normospermia is not present until a bone age of 17 years.

For simplicity, the mean age of onset of puberty in Caucasian boys is 11 years (with 2.5 SD limits at 9–13.5 years of age). Approximately 70% of boys start masturbating in the window of 1 year before to 1 year after the first nocturnal semen emission.

Girl–woman

The first sign of change is the start of the growth spurt, causing for a while a big difference with boys of the same age. However, the female spurt ends also 2 years earlier than in boys. The second change is the breast development (induced by oestrogens) and the growth of pubic and axillary hair (induced by androgens from both ovaries and adrenals). Androgens are not 'male hormones'! Women need testosterone too (for instance, for sexual desire, to fall in love, for arousability, for mood and for muscular strength). Gradually a hormonal cycling pattern develops and the first menses appear (menarche) within the beginning anovulatory cycles. The hormones also cause growth of external genitalia, mons pubis fat and adaptation of the vaginal epithelium with a decrease in the vaginal pH.

Till the start of puberty, boys and girls have the same risk for depression, but from the start of puberty, females have nearly a twice bigger risk (probably the result of lower androgens and the influence of hormonal cycling). The normal range of pubertal onset, in which 95% of girls enter Tanner stage 2, lays between age 8 and 13. This onset is affected by many factors including race, birthweight and maternal age.

The age period at which girls start masturbating is extended over many more years than in boys. Having the first orgasm before puberty happened in 12% of the girls and even at an earlier age than in boys. This could be the result of the androgen increase from the adrenarche.

Further reading

Bancroft, J. (2009) *Human Sexuality and Its Problems*, 3rd edn. Churchill-Livingstone, London, pp. 20–54.

Brizendine, L. (2006) *The Female Brain*. Morgan Road Books, New York.

Brizendine, L. (2010) *The Male Brain*. Morgan Road Books, New York.

Hyde, J.S. (2005) The Gender Similarities Hypothesis. *American Psychologist*, **60**, 581–592.

Tanner, J.M. (1981) *A History of the Study of Human Growth*. Cambridge University Press, Cambridge, MA, pp. 286–298.

CHAPTER 3

Anatomy and Physiology in the Male

Roy J. Levin

Porterbrook clinic, Sheffield, UK

OVERVIEW

- Male foetal sexual development involves the formation of the androgen-secreting testes by the Y sex-linked chromosome that promotes the transformation of the Wolffian ducts into the epididymis, vas deferens and seminal vesicles and the masculinization of the genital tubercle into the penis and scrotum
- Renewed androgen secretion at puberty continues the masculinization by growth of the primary and secondary sex characteristics
- Sexual arousal mechanisms consist of excitation, erection, emission, ejaculation and orgasm in the sexual cycle phases of desire, excitation, orgasm and resolution (DEOR)
- Erection is the product of relaxation of the smooth muscle of the arteries (by vasoactive intestinal peptide (VIP)) and of the cavernosus sinuses (by nitric oxide (NO)) increasing blood flow into these spaces, their expansion then compresses the venous drainage trapping blood in the penis under pressure
- After ejaculation, a post-ejaculation refractory period occurs which inhibits further sexual arousal, its duration increasing from minutes to hours with ageing.

Introduction

In the limited space allocated, only a brief summary of the major features of the anatomy and physiology of male sexual arousal can be accomplished. More details can be found in Chapter 2 and from the further reading section.

Fetal genital development

In the human embryo, a male Wolffian duct system and a female Mullerian duct system are present while both male and female external genitalia are derived from the common genital tubercle. The Y-linked SRY and seven other genes differentiate the male foetal testis from the indifferent ovotestis. This then secretes the anti-Mullerian factor that regresses the Mullerian ducts. In the

presence of androgens secreted by the embryonic testis, starting at weeks 7–8, the Wolffian ducts are stabilized and differentiated into the epididymis, vas deferens and seminal vesicle while the genital tubercle is masculinized into the scrotum and penis. By week 10, the embryo is now designated as the foetus, the glans penis and scrotum have developed. The testes do not begin to descend before 26 weeks, then take until week 32 before they enter the scrotum by their attachment to the gubernaculum muscle. At birth, there is a short peak of testicular secretion which then falls to the low levels of the prepuberal state. The penis is about 4 cm long and there is little growth until puberty.

Puberty

At puberty, which occurs around years 11–13, the testes once again produce a rising level of testosterone which causes the development and growth of various tissues due to their possessing androgen receptors. These include the penis, scrotum, testes, prostate, seminal vesicles (see Figure 3.1), larynx, pelvic striated musculature, long bones, sebaceous skin glands and pubic, facial and axillary hair. The immature boy develops the secondary male characteristics over 5–6 years during adolescence (years 13–19) and has nocturnal emissions of semen (wet dreams). The production of spermatozoa that can fertilize a female occurs during adolescence.

Functional anatomy of the adult genitalia

The penis

The adult penis, when flaccid, is the male urinary conduit but when transformed by the erectile process becomes a penetrative sexual organ. The structures that create this transformation are two parallel 'cylindrical chambers' (*corpora cavernosae*) on either side of the urethra which are separately sheathed by a 2-mm thick membrane, the *tunica albuginea* (Figures 3.2 and 3.4).

A separate third 'cylindrical chamber' lying underneath and around the urethra (*corpora spongiosum*) extends and terminates with the penile glans. A membrane (*Buck's fascia*) covers the cylinders holding them together, and it is covered by a thinner one (*Colles fascia*). The penile arterial blood supply is primarily through the hypogastric artery which gives a branch described as the internal pudendal artery that itself branches forming the bulbourethral, dorsal and cavernosal arteries. The blood is drained

ABC of Sexual Health, Third Edition. Edited by Kevan Wylie.
© 2015 John Wiley & Sons, Ltd. Published 2015 by John Wiley & Sons, Ltd.

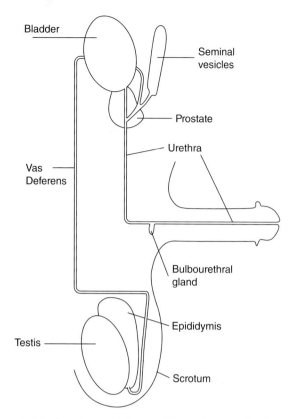

Figure 3.1 A schematic sagittal diagram of the adult male genitourinary tract (not to scale)

from the penis by superficial, intermediate and deep veins finally leading into the femoral vein.

The innervation of the penis is complex having both autonomic (sympathetic and parasympathetic) and somatic (motor and sensory) nerves. The former are the cavernous nerves that enter the corporae cavernosa and spongiosum and derive from neurons in the spinal cord and peripheral ganglia. They supply the smooth muscles of the corpora and mediate erection and detumescence. The somatic nerves primarily serve sensation and the contraction of the ischiocavernosus and bulbocavernosus striated muscles. The latter is a bipennnate structure (see Figure 3.3). The most sensitive parts of the penis are the coronal edge of the glans and the frenulum, and the shaft is the least sensitive. In uncircumcised males, the ridges of the foreskin that covers the glans contain neural sensory end organs; these are lost in the circumcised male.

The four E's of male sexual arousal

These are:

1 *Excitation* – sexual arousal activated by sight, sound, touch, taste, smell and fantasy.
2 *Erection* – in full erection, the penis is rigid and cannot be bent; if it can, it is just tumescent (swollen).
3 *Emission* – movement of genital fluids, secretions and sperm into the prostatic urethra by contractions of smooth muscle mediated by adrenergic innervation in capsules surrounding the testes,

prostate and seminal vesicles and in the ducts of the epididymis and vas deferens.

4 *Ejaculation* – ejection of the semen along the urethra is mediated by peristalsis of the smooth muscle and finally 5–30 powerful expulsive, clonic contractions of the bulbocavernosus striated muscle (see previous section and Figure 3.3), the ischiocavernosus muscle is not involved. The expulsive contractions reduce in frequency, force and pleasure over the duration of ejaculation. If there are no contractions of the striated muscle, then the release of semen is a dribbling one and little pleasure is experienced. After ejaculation, most males cannot immediately have another erection, ejaculation and orgasm. This period is known as the Post Ejaculation Refractory Time (*PERT*). PERT increases with age, lasting from minutes in young adults to hours or more in older men. Although orgasm is usually experienced at ejaculation the two mechanisms are actually independent.

Features of sexual excitation and arousal in males

A number of physical changes occur when males become significantly sexually aroused, these include:

1 increases in respiration (breathing rate can go from basal 12–14 up to 40 min^{-1})
2 increases in heart rate (changing up to 180 beats/min) and blood pressure (systolic increases up to 180 mmHg)
3 nipple erection (in 50–60% of males)
4 increases in genital blood flow creating an erect penis.

Mechanism of erection – converting the flaccid urinary to the sexually erect penis

It has taken over 400 years of conjecture and study to finally unravel the mechanism of penile erection. The early concept proposed, first by Varolius in 1573 and supported later by De Graaf (1668), that the pelvic muscles ischiocavernosus and bulbocavernosus contracted and squeezed off the venous drainage was still endorsed by many recent descriptions but definitive empirical studies in 1990 showed that penile erection occurred without the necessity of pelvic muscular contractions. The mechanism involves three basic features:

1 the vasodilatation of the arteries supplying the penis mainly by the neurotransmitter VIP; this allows increased blood to enter the cavernosal spaces of the two corpora cavernosae.
2 relaxation of the corpora cavernosal smooth musculature mainly by the local release of NO facilitating the entry of blood at near arterial pressure. The activity of its sympathetic nervous innervation is also inhibited.
3 the *veno-occlusive* mechanism is the occlusion of the draining subtunical veins by the filling up of the cavernosal spaces with blood which push up against the unyielding membrane of the tunica albuginea squeezing the veins shut because they obliquely traverse the albuginea (see Figure 3.4). Thus, blood is virtually trapped in the penis.

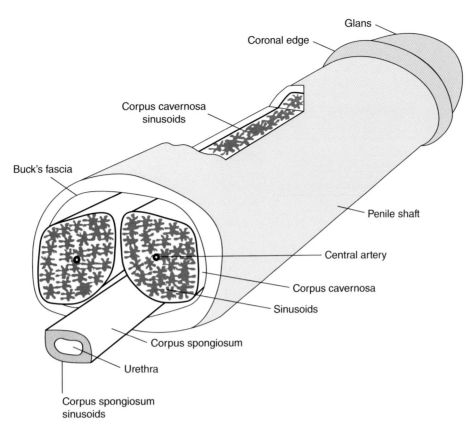

Figure 3.2 A schematic representation of an erect circumcised penis. The paired corpora cavernosa run parallel along the shaft surrounded by the membranous tunica albuginea while underneath the corpora spongiosum is fitted around the urethra and starting as the penile bulb (not shown but see Figure 3.3) and terminates as the penile glans

The corpora spongiosum is not involved in erection as in rare cases of its cancer it can be dissected from the penis without losing the ability of erection. Its filling is to a much lower blood pressure than the corpora cavernosa congruent with its function of protecting the urethra from closure by the expanding cavernosae and creation of the soft cap of the glans acting as a protective shock absorber for the penis and female genitalia during vigorous thrusting.

What keeps the penis flaccid?

A permanent erection would be an obvious embarrassment in everyday life so how is the penis kept flaccid? The major mechanism is the sympathetic nervous supply which continuously releases noradrenaline at it nerve endings that activate the α_1-adrenoreceptors on the smooth muscles of the corpora cavernosae causing them to contract preventing blood from entering the cavernosal spaces. Interestingly, rare cases of the congenital absence of the enzyme dopamine-β-hydroxylase that is essential for the manufacture of noradrenaline do not have permanent erections (*priapism*). It is thought that other vasoconstrictor agents such as endothelins, thromboxanes, prostaglandins and angiotensin all present in the penile tissues act as back-ups for the absent adrenergic supply.

Orgasm

A working definition of male orgasm is 'a variable, transient peak sensation of intense pleasure creating an altered state of consciousness usually concomitant with involuntary rhythmic contractions of pelvic striated muscles and ejection of semen'. Once the mechanism for ejaculation is activated, males feel this point as the moment of 'ejaculatory inevitability', and it cannot be stopped and runs to completion. For most men the first orgasm is usually the most pleasurable. Orgasm causes the release of the hormones oxytocin, prolactin and vasopressin (antidiuretic hormone), but despite being studied for years, their full sexual functions are still surprisingly *sub judice*. It activates the immune system increasing the natural killer cells (characterised by their CD (cluster of differentiation) cell surface molecules identifying and standardizing the leucocytes), higher frequencies reduce prostate cancer and increase longevity (by 50%). Orgasm usually arises from either coitus or masturbation but it can be activated by the stimulation of the prostate gland via the rectum. There have not been any empirical studies of such orgasms but anecdotal reports claim they feel different being 'deeper, more intense and lasting longer'.

The phases of sexual arousal

This sequence was characterized in text and graphically by Masters and Johnson as Excitement, Plateau, Orgasm and Resolution (known by the acronym the *EPOR* model) and for many years stayed unchallenged. More recently, research has shown that the EPOR model needed updating. It is now replaced by the addition of a Desire phase (D-phase) and the amalgamation of the superfluous

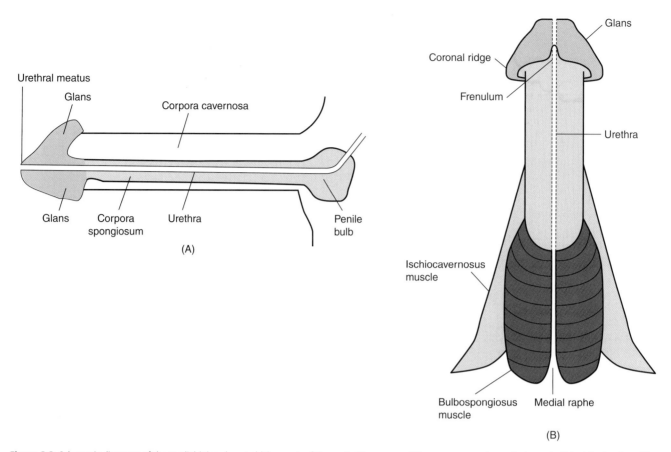

(A)

(B)

Figure 3.3 Schematic diagrams of the medial (A) and ventral (B) aspects of the penis. The course of the corpus spongiosum is shown in (A) while the dispositions of the ischiocavernosus and bulbocavernosus striated muscles are shown in (B). The latter is a bipennate structure with its medial raphe and two rows of muscle fibers facing in opposite diagonal directions; this gives forceful contractions for ejaculation but with restricted movement. The frenulum and coronal edge of the glans are illustrated (see text for details)

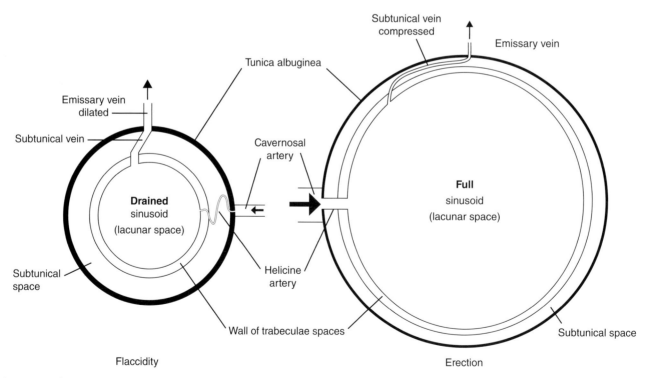

Flaccidity

Erection

Figure 3.4 A diagrammatic illustration of the corpora cavernosal mechanism of erection of the penis (see text for details). The size of the arrows is an indication of the amount of blood flow into and from the vessels involved

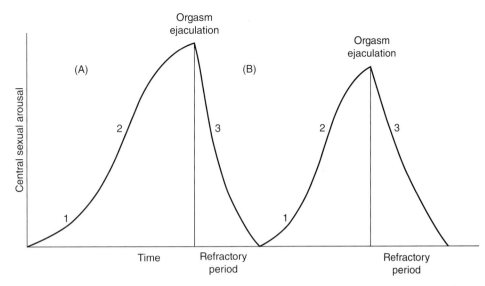

Figure 3.5 A graphic 'cusp' representation of the sexual response cycle in the male during two serial sexual scenarios. Cusp systems have a sudden change caused by a smooth acceleration characterized mathematically by Catastrophe theory. Orgasm is an example of a 'cusp catastrophe' where behaviour is smooth up to the cusp the system then trips over into a completely different behaviour and orgasm occurs. In the first scenario (A) a desire phase (1) precedes the excitement phase (2) and the increasing central sexual arousal reaches a cusp that initiates ejaculation and orgasm. There is then a subsequent resolution (3) back to the basal level. During this resolution phase (3) there is a refractory period (post orgasmic refractory time, PERT) when an immediate further erection/orgasm cannot occur. A subsequent sexual arousal (B), after the ending of the PERT, has the same sequences as the previous but as shown in the diagram the central sexual arousal, thus pleasure, is usually less than the first (see text for details)

Plateau phase into the Excitation phase creating a *DEOR* model. The original graphic depiction of the EPOR model for the male contained some overlooked errors and a more accurate presentation is shown in Figure 3.5.

Brain imaging

The brain is the site of the activation and control of sexual arousal. Brain imaging during ejaculation and orgasm has been undertaken using 'functional magnetic resonance imaging' (*fMRI*) and the tongue-twisting 'blood oxygen level dependent positron emission tomography' (*BOLD-PET*). Rather than a single site for arousal and orgasm, imaging shows multiple site co-activation, some areas become activated some deactivated and some unchanged. The details are beyond the scope of this chapter but can be found in the references and further reading. Unfortunately, different groups have not used comparable experimental designs and data handling so as yet a consensus of brain site activation/inhibition cannot be presented. It is suggested that a main feature of orgasm is the decrease in activity at the cortical level creating behavioural disinhibition allowing dissolution of body boundaries and merging of lovers.

Further reading

Bancroft, J. (2009) *Human Sexuality and Its Problems*, 3rd edn. Churchill Livingstone, Elsevier, Edinburgh.

Georgiadis, J.R., Reinders, A.A., van der Graaf, F.H. *et al.* (2007) Brain activation during human male ejaculation revisited. *Neuroreport*, **18**, 553–557.

Georgiadis, J.R. & Kringlebach, M.L. (2012) The human sexual response cycle: neuroimaging evidence linking sex to other pleasures. *Progress in Neurobiology*, **98**, 48–81.

Georgiadis, J.R., Kringlebach, M.L. & Pfaus, J.G. (2012) Sex for fun: a synthesis of human and animal neurobiology. *Nature Reviews. Urology*, **9**, 486–498.

Levin, R.J. (2005) The mechanisms of human ejaculation- a critical analysis. *Sexual and Relationship Therapy*, **20**, 123–137.

Levin, R.J. (2007) Sexual activity, health and well-being – the beneficial roles of coitus and masturbation. *Sexual and Relationship Therapy*, **22**, 135–148.

Levin, R.J. (2008) Critically revisiting aspects of the human sexual response cycle of Masters and Johnson, correcting errors and suggesting modifications. *Sexual and Relationship Therapy*, **23**, 393–399.

Levin, R.J. (2009) Revisiting post-ejaculation refractory time- what we know and what we don't know in males and females. *Journal of Sexual Medicine*, **6**, 2376–2389.

Masters, W.H. & Johnson, V.E. (1966) *Human Sexual Response*. Little, Brown & Company, Boston, MA.

Tajkarimi, K. & Burnett, A.L. (2011) The role of genital nerve afferents in the physiology of sexual response and pelvic floor function. *Journal of Sexual Medicine*, **8**, 1299–1312.

Thabet, S.M. (2013) New findings and concepts about the G-spot in normal and absent vagina: precautions possibly needed for preservation of the G-spot and sexuality during surgery. *Journal of Obstetrical and Gynaecological Research*, **39**, 1338–1346.

CHAPTER 4

Anatomy and Physiology in the Female

Roy J. Levin

Porterbrook clinic, Sheffield, UK

OVERVIEW

- Female foetal sexual development involves conversion of the Mullerian ducts into the vagina, cervix, uterus and oviducts with the clitoris and labia developing from the genital tubercle
- Vaginal lubrication, a plasma transudate, allows painless coitus and occurs automatically in response to visual and tactile stimulation
- Coitus creates a multisite sexual stimulus involving the clitoris, periurethral glans, labia, G-spot, Halban's fascia and urethra
- Females are multi-orgasmic as they normally do not ejaculate fluid, so do not have a post-orgasmic refractory period
- Orgasm is not involved in reproduction by facilitating sperm transport either by delivering increased numbers or their rate of transport.

Introduction

In the limited space allocated, only a brief summary of the major features of the anatomy and physiology of female sexual arousal can be accomplished. More details can be found in Chapter 2 and from the further reading section.

Foetal genital development

In the absence of the Y sex chromosome (the female is XX), the foetal ovotestis (indifferent gonad) develops as an ovary under the influence of four genes. The male Wolffian duct system regresses with the lack of foetal androgen secretion and the female Mullerian duct system defaults to the development of the vagina, cervix, uterus and oviducts. The clitoris, labia majora and minora develop from the genital tubercle.

Puberty

Girls enter puberty between 8 and 13 years. The ovaries grow and secrete oestrogens, the main stimulus for the growth of breasts (thelarche), uterus, vagina and labia. Androgens from the adrenal

glands (adrenarche) activate the growth of pubic (pubarche) and axillary hair. Menarche (initiation of menstruation) begins around 12–13 years, while the ovaries start to ovulate after 6–9 months. By age 16, most girls have reached adult size and body shape and are menstruating and ovulating regularly.

Functional anatomy of the adult female genitalia

The clitoris and vestibular bulbs

The clitoris has only one function when it is stimulated, the induction of sexual pleasure leading to orgasm. It is composed of a glans, shaft and paired internal crura. Like the penis, it is an androgen-sensitive tissue and will enlarge if androgens are administered (clitoromegaly). The shaft is composed of two corpora cavernosa containing cavernosal sinuses sheathed by a membranous tunica albuginea which, when filled with blood during arousal, make the clitoris tumescent (swollen) but not rigidly erect like the penis as there is no vaso-occlusive mechanism (Figures 4.1 and 4.2). The paired crura also become congested with blood but their function as possible arousing structures is yet to be established. The glans is exceptionally well-innervated with nerve end organs. The vestibular bulbs are paired structures draped over the urethra flanking the vagina with an internal structure similar to the clitoris but are not bounded by a tunica albuginea. While they become engorged during arousal, their structural/functional role has not been definitively characterized.

Periurethral glans

This is the suggested name for the triangular area of the vaginal vestibule around the opening of the urethra (urinary meatus) that is erotically sensitive to frictional stimulation during coitus by the rubbing shaft of the penis (Figure 4.1). A heightened sensitivity may be the reason why some women can experience coital orgasm from just penile vaginal thrusting alone (see Orgasm).

The labia

The labia majora are two cutaneous folds on either side of the vagina stretching from the mons pubis to the perineum and correspond to the male scrotum. During sexual arousal, they become congested

---

ABC of Sexual Health, Third Edition. Edited by Kevan Wylie.
© 2015 John Wiley & Sons, Ltd. Published 2015 by John Wiley & Sons, Ltd.

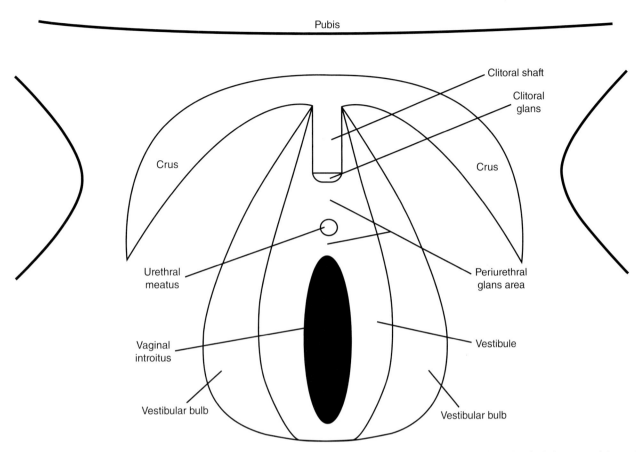

Figure 4.1 A highly schematic diagram of the female pudenda with the labia majora and minora removed for clarity. The periurethral glans area of the vaginal vestibule stretches from underneath the clitoris to the top of the introitus

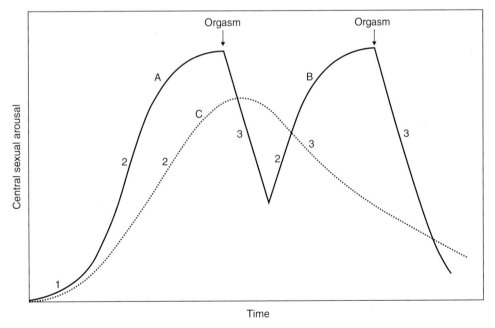

Figure 4.2 A graphic representation of the female sexual response cycles for two scenarios. The first (A) is represented by a cusp system. Cusp systems have a sudden change caused by a smooth acceleration characterized mathematically by Catastrophe theory. Orgasm is an example of a 'cusp catastrophe' where behaviour is smooth up to the cusp, the system then trips over into a completely different behaviour and orgasm occurs. In A (solid line), a desire phase (1) precedes the excitement phase (2) created by sexual stimulation. The rising central sexual arousal reaches a cusp that initiates orgasm and then a partial resolution (3) of the arousal until a further bout of stimulation (2) in B arrests the resolution and a second central arousal reaches the cusp and the induction of a further orgasm. This then induces the subsequent resolution phase (3) that returns the central arousal back to near basal levels. The second scenario (C, dotted line) again has an initial desire phase (1) preceding the excitement phase (2) but this time the central sexual arousal does not reach the level required to activate the orgasm cusp, orgasm does not occur, so the resolution phase (3) takes a considerably longer time to resolve back to basal level

with blood and increase in size some twofold. The labia minora are skin folds of great variation of size and shape found on either side of the vaginal vestibule between the labia majora. Their lateral parts form the hood or prepuce that covers the shaft of the clitoris, while underneath they form its frenulum. They become congested on sexual arousal and increase in size. They are well-innervated along their edges and create pleasurable sexual arousal when stimulated.

The vagina

The adult vagina, the female organ of social fusion, is an elongated S-shaped canal some 9 cm long extending from the posterior fornix (its blind end) to the introitus (entrance) at the vulva in the sexually unstimulated woman who has not given birth (nulliparous). It can be regarded as a potential space with an H- or W-shaped cross-section. It is lined with a stratified squamous epithelium thrown into folds (rugae) that allow great expansion during childbirth and sexual arousal. The epithelium is sensitive to and maintained by oestrogens. Beneath it, is a layer of smooth muscle surrounded by connective tissue (adventitia) containing many blood vessels. The septum between the anterior wall and the bladder has Halban's fascia containing neural end organs that on pressure stimulation can create sexual arousal (Figure 4.3).

The vaginal luminal surface is kept just moist, to prevent adhesion of opposite walls, through plasma transudation into the lumen and subsequent osmotic reabsorption of fluid by a limited lumen-to-blood Na^+ transfer. Increased vaginal lubrication is necessary for painless penile penetration and thrusting during coitus, it is an automatic response to visual and tactile stimulation.

The vaginal blood supply in the unaroused state is limited because a large number of capillaries in its micro-circulation are closed. Local hypoxia and build-up of metabolites cause transient pseudo-random opening and closing of capillaries known as 'vasomotion'. When sexual arousal occurs, the neural innervation to the arterial supply causes vasodilatation through the agency of the neurotransmitter Vasoactive intestinal peptide (VIP) and new capillaries become open. Gradually, vasomotion is greatly reduced until all the capillaries are open and the microcirculation of the vagina is completely vasocongested. This causes a greatly enhanced plasma transudate to leak from the capillaries, pass through the vaginal epithelium onto its surface as increased vaginal lubrication allowing painless penile penetration and thrusting. Cessation of arousal allows vasomotion to return and the osmotic reabsorption of the excess lubrication by the lumen-to-blood Na^+ transfer.

The cervix

This is the neck of the uterus and has a lumen (cervical canal) that allows sperm entry into the uterus and menstrual discharge. Its poor sensory innervation and utero-cervical elevation during arousal indicate its lack of involvement in coital arousal by penile buffeting (Figure 4.3).

The G-spot

The G-spot is a claimed area of the anterior vaginal wall one-third to one-half up from the vaginal introitus that on stimulation rapidly creates arousal to orgasm. It was first described by Ernst Graafenberg in 1950 and since then the topic has been highly contentious with claims and counter claims of its anatomical existence. While women report that stimulation of the anterior vaginal wall is indeed highly arousing, this alone does not prove its presence because there are other features that could be the cause of the arousal (Halban's fascia, urethra, internal clitoral structures). Two reports have described dissections purporting to reveal the G-spot, one only in the single cadaver of an 83-year-old woman, but they differ in structure and genital site. Further studies are essential before a conclusion can be reached.

Orgasm

Although orgasm is the most pleasure available without recourse to drugs, it strangely creates a characteristic 'orgasm face' that looks as if the person is suffering from severe pain. It can occur when asleep, from a variety of non-genital stimuli and even without consensual sexual arousal. Its duration is some 20 seconds (±12, standard deviation) and this is unconnected with subjective feelings of pleasure. At orgasm, the release of the hormones prolactin, oxytocin and vasopressin (antidiuretic hormone) occurs.

The function and the induction of the female orgasm are the foci of controversy. Many speculative roles have been postulated that it represents an evolutionary adaptation to enhance 'reproductive fitness', but as there is no crucial test that can falsify their validity they are likened to the children's 'Just so stories' of how animals obtained their specific anatomies. Despite repeated suggestions in the literature, there is no scientific evidence for its involvement in facilitating sperm transport either in terms of speed or quantity. An often quoted typology identifies two induction sites, that induced by clitoral stimulation and that induced by vaginal stimulation through penile vaginal intercourse (PVI) alone. A few propose that the latter are 'healthier' than those of the former and that women who do

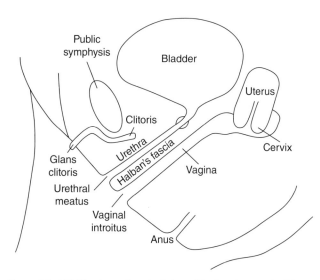

Figure 4.3 A highly schematic sagittal view of the female genitalia (labia majora and minora not shown). The septum between the anterior wall of the vagina and the urethra contains Halban's fascia (see text). A possible site for the controversial G-spot is shown just around the junction of the bladder and urethra

not have PVI orgasms are sexually dysfunctional, but others have criticized the studies and their conclusions.

At orgasm, most women experience pelvic muscular contractions but the function of these and the link between them and pleasure is unknown as voluntary contraction of the muscles does not create pleasure. Uterine contractions also occur but these are not normally perceived. Unlike males, females can have repeated multiple orgasms probably because they rarely ejaculate genital fluids.

Some studies have reported that reflexes causing mainly pelvic muscular contractions can be elicited by distension of the vagina, but the physiological role of these during coitus is yet to be confirmed.

Sexual response cycle

As for the male, the sexual response cycle of Masters and Johnson is now refined from the original EPOR phases (Excitation, Plateau, Orgasm, Resolution) to the DEOR phases (Desire, Excitation, Orgasm, Resolution – see Figure 4.2 for graphical depiction). A further modification for the female is that the D-phase can be split into two, D_1 which is sexual desire created spontaneously (endogenous desire) and D_2 desire created by initiation of sexual arousal (reactive desire) thus giving the D_1D_2EOR model. The underlying neural mechanism creating D_1 is as yet unknown. In the late E-phase, the uterus and the cervix are elevated from the vaginal posterior floor by pelvic muscle contractions and the back of the vagina balloons out. This elevation is crucial for reproduction as it delays the transport of any ejaculated spermatozoa allowing time to become reprogrammed (capacitation) by contact with various secreted male and female genital factors into sperm that can fertilize ova.

Brain imaging

As in the male there is no consensual agreement among investigators as to the specific activity of the brain during arousal to orgasm. One study claims that only one area shows reliable orgasm-related activity while another describes a non-uniform sequence of activity of different brain areas.

Menopause

The cessation of the ovarian secretion of oestrogens brings about the end of menstruation and starts the menopause. All the tissues supported by the hormone (breasts, vagina, cervix, skin) show atrophic changes. Vaginal lubrication is reduced and orgasm is said to be less intense.

Further reading

Bancroft, J. (2009) *Human Sexuality and Its Problems*, 3rd edn. Churchill Livingstone, London.

Georgiadis, J.R. (2011) Exposing orgasm in the brain: a critical eye. *Sexual and Relationship Therapy*, **26**, 342–355.

Goldstein, I., Meston, C.M., Davis, S.R. & Traish, A.M. (2006) *Women's Sexual Function and Dysfunction-Study, Diagnosis and Treatment*. Taylor & Francis, London.

Laan, E. & Rellini, A.H. (2011) Can we treat anorgasmia in women? The challenge to experiencing pleasure. *Sexual and Relationship Therapy*, **26**, 239–341.

Levin, R.J. (2003) Do women gain anything from coitus apart from pregnancy? Changes in the human female genital tract activated by coitus. *Journal of Sex and Marital Therapy*, **29**, 59–69.

Levin, R.J. (2004) An orgasm is … who defines what an orgasm is? *Sex and Relationship Therapy*, **19**, 101–107.

Levin, R.J. & Wylie, K. (2008) Vaginal vasomotion – its appearance, measurement, and usefulness in assessing the mechanisms of vasodilatation. *Journal of Sexual Medicine*, **5**, 377–386.

Levin, R.J. (2008) Critically revisiting aspects of the human sexual response cycle of Masters & Johnson: correcting errors and suggesting modifications. *Sexual and Relationship Therapy*, **23**, 393–399.

Levin, R.J. (2011) Can the controversy about the putative role of the human female orgasm in sperm transport be settled with our current physiological knowledge of coitus? *Journal of Sexual Medicine*, **8**, 1566–1578.

Levin, R.J. (2011) Special issue: the human orgasm. *Sexual and Relationship Therapy*, **16**, 299–402.

Levin, R.J. (2011) The human female orgasm: a critical evaluation of its proposed reproductive functions. *Sexual and Relationship Therapy*, **26**, 301–314.

Levin, R.J. (2012) The deadly pleasures of the clitoris and the condom – a rebuttal of Brody, Costa and Hess (2012). *Sexual and Relationship Therapy*, **27**, 272–295.

Masters, W.H. and Johnson, V.E. (1966) Human Sexual Response. Little, Brown & Company, Boston.

Ostrzenski, A. (2012) G-spot anatomy: a new discovery. *Journal of Sexual Medicine*, **9**, 1355–1359.

Pastor, Z. (2013) Female ejaculation orgasm vs coital incontinence: a systematic review. *Journal of Sexual Medicine*, **10**, 1682–1691.

Prause, N. (2012) A response to Brody, Costa and Hess (2102); theoretical, statistical and construct problems perpetuated in the study of female orgasm. *Sexual and Relationship Therapy*, **27**, 260–271.

Salonia, A., Giraldi, A., Chivers, M.L. *et al.* (2010) Physiology of women's sexual function: basic knowledge and new findings. *Journal of Sexual Medicine*, **7**, 2637–2660.

Thabet, S.M. (2013) New findings and concepts about the G-spot in normal and absent vagina: precautions possibly needed for preservation of the G-spot and sexuality during surgery. *Journal of Obstetrical and Gynaecological Research*, **39**, 1338–1346.

CHAPTER 5

The Sexual History and Formulation

Julie A. Fitter

Porterbrook Clinic, Sheffield Health and Social Care NHS Foundation Trust, Sheffield, UK

> **OVERVIEW**
> - Taking a sexual history and developing a formulation are essential to a good understanding of sexual health and sexual problems
> - Understanding of context, clinician and patient comfort in talking about sexual matters should be considered
> - A biopsychosocial model is recommended to understand and work with sexual difficulties in an integrated way.

Taking a sexual history and developing a formulation are essential to a good understanding of sexual health and sexual problems. They will assist the clinician and their patient(s) in deciding on the best way forward when presented with sexual difficulties. Recent estimations are that between 29% and up to 44% of people will experience a sexual difficulty at some time in their lives (Figure 5.1).

The sexual history

A sexual history is relevant in many clinical specialties, where the people who present might be experiencing sexual and/or relationship difficulties, for example general practice, psychiatry, cardiology, gynaecology, urology, dermatology and endocrinology. Unfortunately, this area is often neglected due to clinician's own discomfort in asking the questions, worries about how, where and when to ask the questions, of whom to ask and what to do with the information that is collected. This can seem increasingly difficult in time pressure practice.

Some things that may be helpful to consider when to take a sexual history are as follows:

- *Context yours and your patients* – Can you give enough time, for instance you could arrange a longer appointment, or time to return; is the consultation in a private area that will not be overheard or interrupted; can you sit away from a desk, or at least align yourself adjacent to your patient rather than sitting behind a desk, which might help both you and your patient to feel less formal and more at ease; would it be possible to include the patient's partner in the consultation? (Figure 5.2)

- *Your own comfort talking about sexual issues* what might make it easier? For example, practice, as well as understanding and working on your own embarrassment or discomfort; diagrams; non-verbal communication, that is, making eye contact, giving enough time and encouragement to speak, active listening, empathy, non-judgmental response; making sure you have shared meanings for any terms used. It may be possible to arrange to observe other clinicians working in psychosexual services, to increase your own confidence in this area and to develop your own questioning and assessment technique.

- *Developing a standard question/patter/assessment tool* considering where this would best fit into your own practice, and possibly writing it into, or including a separate sheet, during your own assessment. Some clinicians find it helpful to have the questions written down, as it may 'validate' asking the questions, as part of the assessment. Consider also starting the interview with a statement such as 'we know that sexual problems are sometimes experienced by people attending this service/with these sort of conditions/taking these medications', which legitimizes taking a sexual history (Figure 5.3).

- *Use of language yours or theirs?* Although it might put patients at ease initially if you are able to hear their own language to describe their problems, and to demonstrate that you are comfortable and not offended by this, it is also helpful to clarify and give some correct anatomical and medical terms, as these will help patients become more confident in discussing their problem with other professionals, as necessary. It may also help to alleviate their embarrassment in talking about sexual and intimate matters in future – which is likely to be greater than that of the clinician, in the majority of cases.

- *Consider carefully why and when you might not feel comfortable in asking these questions* for example to older people, disabled people, young people, people with long-term conditions and people engaging in non-monogamous or non-heterosexual relationships. Discomfort may be based on assumptions about the sort of people who do (or 'should') have sex and may be inaccurate or discriminatory. People can experience sexual difficulties at any time in the lifespan and a sexual relationship may become more or less important at different times in life, which may not necessarily be those we as clinicians would expect.

- *Resources* consider collecting resources to assist you and your patients once you have recorded the sexual history. Useful

ABC of Sexual Health, Third Edition. Edited by Kevan Wylie.
© 2015 John Wiley & Sons, Ltd. Published 2015 by John Wiley & Sons, Ltd.

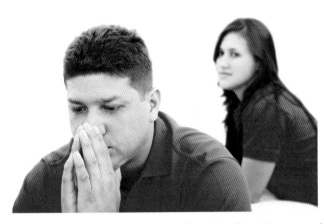

Figure 5.1 Between 29% and up to 44% of people will experience a sexual difficulty at some time in their lives

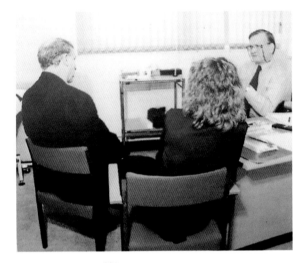

Figure 5.2 Taking a sexual history

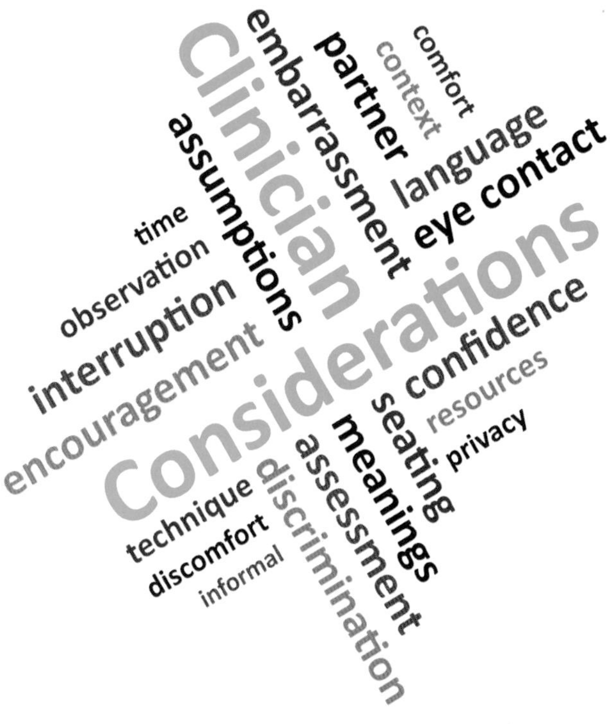

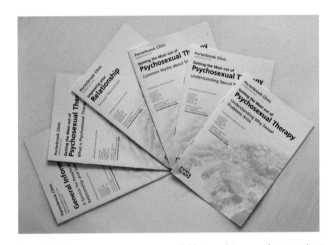

Figure 5.3 Clinician considerations

Figure 5.4 There are many resources available to assist you and your patients

reading material, web sites, information leaflets, organizations and appropriate referral pathways will help build confidence that you are able to signpost patients to relevant pathways, if you are not able to provide this yourself, or within your service or organization (Figure 5.4).

- *Couple or individual assessment* there are pros and cons to inviting individuals alone for assessment rather than with their partner. Seeing an individual alone, before a couple's assessment or couple's therapy, may allow the individual to share information that they may feel inhibited to mention if their partner was present, for example other relationships, sexual behaviours or preferences about which their partner is unaware or about which they feel ashamed, current or previous abuse and feelings about their partner. This is more likely to be problematic if they have not been able to express directly to the partner, for example whether or not they find their partner attractive. However, this should be mediated against the increased value to the assessment of a partner's perspective and information.

Ethical dilemmas can occur if information is shared in an individual assessment that the patient does not want to be disclosed

to the partner, and how the clinician then accommodates this in any further appointments, particularly if this information or couple issues are relevant to the formulation. Seeing a couple together from the outset allows each individual to decide what information to share with the partner and clinician. Even if they do not feel able to share information honestly at the outset, as trust develops, further appointments may lead to building confidence in sharing the information. Sessions can provide a safe place for this to be processed. Seeing a couple together also allows the clinician to gain some insight into how the couple function together and to identify unhelpful patterns of communication or scripts. If these are not attended to in work with couples, benefits are likely to be restricted, along with the tolerance and efficacy of, and commitment to, treatments (Figure 5.5).

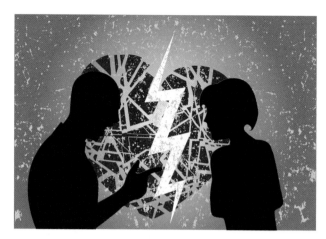

Figure 5.5 Seeing a couple together also allows the clinician to gain some insight into how the couple function together and to identify unhelpful patterns of communication

Items to be included in a sexual history:
Nature and understanding of current sexual problem:

- How patient sees the problem (general description),
- Frequency of sexual interest and desire, including onset and details of any change,
- Ease and frequency of ability to fantasize,
- Process of arousal including for men details of when erections are achieved and maintained, at what percentage of full or partial erection and under what circumstances, for example early morning, with partner, during foreplay and intercourse, during masturbation, during oral sex, using erotica, spontaneous,
- Amount of stimulation needed to become aroused,
- Confidence and frequency in achieving orgasm,
- Whether any difficulties are only related to partner sex or also present during masturbation,
- For men – nature and duration of any ejaculatory problems (rapid, inhibited or delayed or retrograde),
- Detail of any sexual pain – where, when, frequency, duration and type,
- Difficulties with penetration, for example with tampon, finger, penis or during vaginal examination,
- Any factors that make the problem better or worse.

Past and current medical history:

- Chronic and acute conditions,
- Mental health problems,
- Genetic conditions,
- Surgical procedures (including specifically circumcision, vasectomy, hysterectomy and female genital mutilation),
- Family history,
- Cardiovascular risk factors, including smoking, alcohol and hypertension,
- For women details of menstrual and obstetric history, including number of pregnancies and details of these,
- Treatments for any of these.

Past and current sexual history:

- Details of sex education,
- Messages learned about sex,
- Age of first sexual experience,
- Details of significant sexual experiences,
- Number of sexual partners,
- Sexual orientation and comfort with this,
- Details of specified or unspecified paraphilic or fetishistic disorders or behaviours,
- Any history of sexual abuse/trauma and whether this is something that has been addressed, if necessary,
- If patient or their partner has any other sexual difficulties.

Gender history:

- Comfort in gender role now and in the past and any associated dysphoria,
- History of cross dressing and any arousal associated with this,
- Feelings of being in the wrong body and wanting to be the opposite gender to that assigned at birth,
- Any desire to transition away from the assigned gender,
- Any arousal at the thought of themselves as the opposite gender.

Past and current relationship history:

- Number of significant relationships,
- Any experiences of difficult relationships,
- How long relationships have lasted,
- Duration of current relationship,
- Circumstances of getting together,
- How relationship is seen in terms of communication, commitment, negotiation and resolving conflict,
- Whether they find partner attractive.

Medication:

- Past and current use of prescribed and non-prescribed agents,
- Including off licence or herbal supplements and performance enhancing steroids.

Formulation

A clinical formulation (or case formulation) is a theoretically based explanation or conceptualization of the information obtained from a clinical assessment. It offers a hypothesis about the cause and nature of the presenting problems and is considered an alternative approach to the more categorical approach of psychiatric diagnosis. In clinical practice, formulations are used to communicate a hypothesis and provide a framework to develop the most suitable treatment approach. Following a sexual history, it is helpful in understanding mixed aetiology sexual problems, and is well employed when integrating medical and psychological approaches.

A biopsychosocial model (Figure 5.6) is useful in considering the sexual history and formulation. This holistic approach takes into account biological, psychological, social, cultural, relationship and educational factors which may affect sexual health and function.

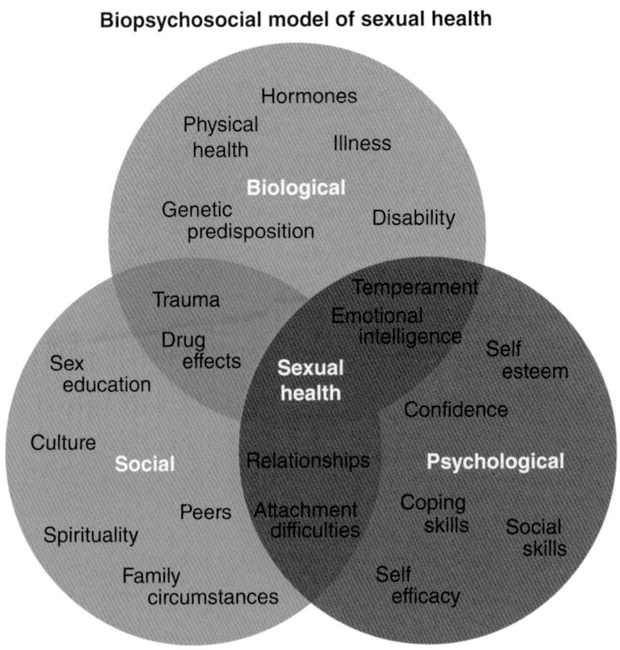

Biopsychosocial model of sexual health

Figure 5.6 Biopsychosocial model

These can be further understood in relation to predisposing, precipitating and maintaining factors, originally described by Hawton (1985), but remaining relevant nearly 30 years hence.

Predisposing factors are the long-term experiences that might influence sexual thoughts, feelings and behaviours, for example the family of upbringing views of sex, specifically restricted views; how sex and intimacy were addressed during early life experience; secretive, hurried or shameful early masturbatory development and how these were interpreted via cultural or faith learning experiences. They might also include chronic conditions, childhood sexual abuse or attachment difficulties. In psychotherapy terms these might be best addressed via a psychodynamic or exploratory approach, and how these have shaped a person's sexual development and unconscious processes.

Precipitating factors are those which might be understood as 'triggers' and are likely to have occurred just before the onset of the problem. A recent medical diagnosis, change in medication, bereavement, job loss, life stressors, relationship change, domestic abuse or family transitions would be examples of these factors. When working therapeutically, these factors tend to lend themselves well (but not exclusively) to the cognitive-behavioural approach.

Maintaining factors are those patterns of interaction and/or behaviour that influence the problem and 'keep it going'. These might be displayed as communication difficulties in couples, sexual boredom, relationship conflict, depression in one partner, cognitive interference, for example in negative and automatic thoughts, and in making assumptions of others. The systemic model of therapy is a useful way of understanding and working with these factors, when one way of creating change in the problem might be in changing the unhelpful patterns or scripts. This way of working is particularly

suited to working with couples, and can be helpful in addressing couple's script problems and the adoption of unhelpful roles when involved in intimate relationships, for example parent/child or carer/patient.

Whilst it is accepted that biological, organic or medical factors are important in understanding the things that might adversely affect sexual function, for example cardiovascular disease, chronic conditions such as diabetes or multiple sclerosis, or hormonal imbalances, these need to be considered alongside other issues. Psychological factors are also relevant in understanding and working with sexual difficulties, for example performance anxiety, sexual myths, automatic negative thoughts, body image, sexual self-confidence issues, anxiety, inaccurate sex education and poor or incomplete understanding of sexual function.

In the current climate of increasing availability of physical and medical approaches to treating sexual difficulties, there is a danger amongst the public and clinicians of looking for a 'quick fix'. Clinical treatments are likely be more efficacious, efficient, better tolerated and understood by patients and their partners if they are used appropriately and relevantly integrated with psychological interventions (Wylie *et al.* 2003). This should be guided by a good sexual history and formulation, to offer treatments as clinically indicated, integrated with sex education, challenging myths, improving understanding, addressing relationship difficulties, attending to unresolved trauma or attachment difficulties, opportunities to try alternative ways of being sexual and normalizing the variety of sexual response in today's increasingly electronic, overwhelming and sometimes unhelpful availability of information about sex.

Items to be included in a sexual history adapted from the Porterbrook Clinic Female and Male Sex History Data Collections sheets. Copies/information available on request from: porterbrook@shsc.nhs.uk.

Further reading

Baker, C.D. (1993) A cognitive-behavioural model for the formulation and treatment of sexual dysfunction. In: Ussher, J.M. & Baker, C.D. (eds), *Psychological Perspectives on Sexual Problems*. Routledge, London, pp. 110–128.

Bancroft, J. (2009) *Human Sexuality and It's Problems*. (3rd edition). Churchill Livingstone. Elsevier, Europe.

Basson, R. (2003) Biopsychosocial models of women's sexual response: applications to management of 'desire disorders'. *Sexual and Relationship Therapy*, **18** (**1**), 107–115.

Bhugra, D. & Colombini, G. (2013) Sexual dysfunction: classification and assessment. *Royal College of Psychiatrists Advances in Psychiatric Treatment*, **19**, 48–55.

Goldstein, I., Meston, C.M., Davis, S. & Traish, A. (2006) *Women's Sexual Function and Dysfunction*. Taylor & Francis, London.

Hawton, K. (1985) *Sex Therapy: A Practical Guide*. Oxford Medical Pulbications. Oxford.

Hinchliff, S., Gott, M. (2011). Seeking medical help for sexual concerns in mid and later life: a review of the literature. *Journal of Sex Research*, **48**, 106–117.

Laumann, E.O., Nicolosi, A., Glasser, D.B., *et al.* (2005) Sexual problems among men and women aged 40-80 years. *International Journal of Impotence Research*, **17**, 39–57.

Lebow, J.L., Chambers, A.L., Christensen, A., Johnson, S.M. (2012) Research on the treatment of couple distress. *Journal of Marital and Family Therapy*, **38**(1), 145–168.

Leiblum, S.R. (2007) *Principles and Practice of Sex Therapy*, 5th edn. The Guilford Press, New York.

McCabe, M., Althof, S.E., Assaillian, P. *et al.* (2010) Psychological and interpersonal dimensions of sexual function and dysfunction. *Journal of Sexual Medicine*, **7**, 327–336.

Moreria, E., Glasser, D. *et al.* (2005) Sexual behaviour for sexual problems: the global study of sexual attitudes and behaviours. *International Journal of Clinical Practice*, **59**, 6–16.

Wylie, K.R., Hallam-Jones, R. & Walters, S. The potential benefit of vacuum devices augmenting psychosexual therapy for erectile dysfunction: a randomised controlled trial. *Journal of Sex & Marital Therapy 2003*, **29**(3), 227–236.

CHAPTER 6

The Clinical Examination of Men and Women

David Goldmeier

Imperial College London, St Marys Hospital, London, UK

OVERVIEW

- The aim of the examination is to gather diagnostic information, adding to what has been already obtained in the history
- The examiner should have at least reasonable knowledge of genital anatomy
- Details of what will take place should be discussed with patient before the examination
- Every effort should be made to examine the patient at some stage, but discussion with the patient will inform the examiner when, where and who should undertake this
- The examination should be conducted at a pace acceptable to the patient – with continuous monitoring of their emotional and pain status
- The examiner should make it quite clear that the examination can be halted at any point if the patient wishes
- Wherever possible, a chaperone should be present.

Box 6.1 **Sexual health in general practice**

About two-thirds of both men and women in the UK who seek help for sexual problems go to their GP. However, GPs and their practice nurses construe sexual health problems as 'opening up a can of worms', in that these are complex and sensitive issues which require time and expertise to handle.

Mercer *et al.*, 2003; Gott, 2004.

Introduction

Examination of the patient with sexual problems may be embarrassing or even distressing for the patient. However, if it is undertaken with adequate knowledge of local anatomy and physiology, and with sympathy and compassion it is likely to be diagnostically and therapeutically useful. Examination should always be at the patient's pace, with continuous monitoring of the patient for signs of distress. Details of local genital examination for men and women are described.

The aim of the physical examination of men and women who have sexual problems is primarily to gather diagnostic information, building on the information gathered during history taking. Very often it will also yield therapeutic fruit. It almost always involves examination of the genitalia. It is likely to be a routine and regular activity for the health care practitioner (HCP) (Box 6.1). For the patient it may an event that is at best somewhat embarrassing, but in others it will be feared and cause great distress, pain or shame. Spending a few moments before the examination (better still a few minutes at the start of each day), empathizing compassionately how

the patient might be feeling about the examination will help make the examining HCP more a sympathetic ally rather than an invader of privacy and dignity.

The examining HCP might also wish to look at their own ideas and feelings of the genitalia. There may be cultural or religious reasons as to why they are uncomfortable about such an examination. These might be discussed with a more senior and experienced colleague. It should go without saying that the HCP has at least some understanding of the organic and psychological aspects of sexual medicine, as well as being reasonably informed about the relevant genital anatomy and physiology.

The patient should be allowed to undress in privacy and with dignity. The examination should not be rushed and should be undertaken at a rate the patient can handle physically and emotionally. In patients who have a history of sexual assault or who are phobic, the examination may have to be deferred for some time. It should be done in warm and comfortable surroundings with maximal privacy. Phones (HCW and patient) should be switched off or silenced, and knocks on doors ignored. The patient should understand from the outset that they have control of what is being done and can signal at any time for the process to cease (e.g. if they are anxious or in pain). Before the examination, the HCW should explain as clearly as possible what will be done. Some patients, particularly women greatly appreciate seeing what is going on by means of a large hand-held mirror. A good light is very important. The examination should be as meticulous and methodical as the patient will allow. The HCW should be inspecting the relevant area, but should also be constantly checking the patient's psychological and physical response to what is happening by looking at their facial expression and movement and lie of the hands and the legs.

ABC of Sexual Health, Third Edition. Edited by Kevan Wylie.
© 2015 John Wiley & Sons, Ltd. Published 2015 by John Wiley & Sons, Ltd.

Another important consideration is the need for an appropriate chaperone. *about here* The patient should be given a choice of the sex of the examiner, although ideally there should be continuity between the person taking the history and doing the examination. See GMC guidance below (Box 6.2). This will be particularly pertinent in women say from Muslim backgrounds. Where the patient has limited movement, for example arthritis, due consideration should be given when setting up the patient for examination.

Most attention will be given to the genital area, but sometimes areas distant from this may need to be examined. Examples of this are general neurological examination in women with vulval pain (with an emphasis on the pelvic and genital areas), cardiovascular system in men with suspected arteriosclerotic erectile dysfunction (e.g. looking for peripheral leg pulses and taking blood pressure), or presence of facial and genital hair in men with low sexual desire.

Men

Penis

The penis may be inspected with the man standing up. Any significant curvature should be noted. In the non-erect state, it is between 5 and 10 cm long. However, if the patient is anxious or there is fat around the pubic area it may appear smaller. The penis should be examined in a methodical manner, to include inspection and where appropriate palpation of the glans and meatus, coronal and subcoronal areas, the outer foreskin where present and the dorsal (corpora cavernosa) and ventral shaft (corpus spongiosum). Particular note should be made of the presence of indurated or hard corporeal areas (Peyronie's disease), dermatoses (balanitis), papules (e.g. warts) or ulceration. The man should be asked to retract his foreskin where present. His emotional response to this as well as the appearance of the retracted foreskin should be noted. The frenular area should also be examined looking particularly for fibrosis and fissuring with pain on retraction. Size and tenderness of the dorsal vein should be noted.

Testes

The testes should be smooth and about 4 cm long (15–25 ml in volume), with the epididymis posteriorly and inferiorly feeling soft and less smooth than the globe of the testis. The spermatic cord can be just felt between the testes and groin. Cysts of the epididymis and spermatic cord are common and almost always benign. The presence of varicocoeles and inguinal hernias should be noted.

Prostate and pelvic floor

The prostate should be palpated in men with erectile dysfunction and urinary symptoms, men with secondary premature ejaculation or genital or peri-genital pain. The size of the gland varies but it should be smooth and symmetrical and not significantly tender or painful on digital pressure. The median groove should be present and any hard or irregular areas noted. The pelvic floor tone and degree of tenderness on palpation should also be noted.

Neurological examination in men

A focused neurological examination should be undertaken if the history suggests a neurological cause for their sexual problem. Multiple sclerosis or diabetic or alcoholic neuropathy may underpin erectile dysfunction or delayed ejaculation. Sensory examination should be focused between the lower inguinal area and anal region to include the genitalia. Lower limb motor, sensory and reflex assessment may also be informative.

The bulbocavernosus reflex – squeezing the penile glans to elicit anal contraction – tests the integrity of the spinal reflex via the pudendal nerve (Boxes 6.3 and 6.4).

Female

Physical examination of the genitalia may not be necessary for all female sexual dysfunction issues, but when undertaken can often be very reassuring for the woman, even where pathology is unlikely to be found, for example in women with low sexual desire.

Box 6.3 **The pudendal nerve**

The Pudendal nerve provides sensory information from lower mons pubis, clitoris, perineum and anus. Local muscle contractions at orgasm are also innervated by pudendal nerve (contraction of bulbo-cavernosus and ischiocavernosus), as are clitoral erectile responses. Bladder and anal sphincters are supplied by motor branches.

Box 6.4 **Autonomic innervation of the genitalia**

The anogenital and bladder areas have dual innervation.

1 From the T11-L3 via the hypogastric and pelvic innervation. This is mainly sympathetic and controls emission (depositing semen in posterior urethra rather than ejaculation).
2 From S2,3,4 via pudendal, perineal and dorsal penile nerves. These send sensory information from the penis, scrotum, perineum and anal areas. They also provides motor innervation to the bulbocavernosus and ischiocavernosus muscles, cavernosal vessels and anal and bladder sphincters.

Physical examination may not be appropriate early on in the management of the woman. Thus where the complaint is difficult or painful vaginal penetration, examination is mandatory (differential diagnosis vaginismus, provoked vestibulodynia or other local pathology), but the patient should be in no doubt that it will be done where and when anxiety is at a manageable level. Behavioural desensitization may have to precede local genital examination in women who are phobic or express disgust at the idea of genital examination. Where past sexual assault has resulted in post-traumatic stress disorder, extended specialist psychological intervention may have to precede the genital examination. However, the examination may be very reassuring, for example showing the women that pelvic floor tenderness produced by gentle digital palpation of these contracted muscles may reproduce the pain she develops at intercourse.

External genitalia

The labia majora and minora should be carefully inspected for lesions, for example dermatoses such as eczema or lichen sclerosus or infections such as genital herpes. The appearance of the vulvar vestibule, for example erythema should be noted, as well as local neurological testing of this area – see below. Bartholin's glands and the orifice of duct leading from them should be noted as should the posterior fourchette (episiotomy scars), the hymeneal ring and hymeneal remnants (and any associated redness or tenderness). The level of oestrogenization of the vulva should be noted.

Internal genitalia

It may be appropriate to undertake a vaginal examination, where the appearance of the vaginal walls and exudate should be noted. Like-wise, the cervix should be assessed for ectopy, IUD threads and the degree and type of discharge, for example mucopurulent might suggest gonorrhoea or chlamydia. Where appropriate, the pubic area, clitoris, clitoral hood, urethral orifice and perianal areas should be examined. A bimanual examination might be considered, particularly if there are complaints of deep dyspareunia.

Neurological examination in women

This should be undertaken according to symptomatology assessing relevant areas from the lower inguinal area to the anus including the external genitalia, including the lower limbs if appropriate. Particular attention should be paid to presence of allodynia (pain on touch), hyperpathia (pain on very light touch) and hyperaesthesia in the vulvar vestibule.

Further reading

General Medical Council (2013) Intimate examinations and chaperones. Online http://www.gmc-uk.org/Intimate_examinations_and_chaperones .pdf_51449880.pdf, March 2013.

Gott, M. (2004) "Opening a can of worms": GP and practice nurses barriers to talking about sexual health in primary care. *Family Practice*, **21**, 528–536.

Mercer, C.H., Fenton, K.A., Johnson, A.M. *et al.* (2003) Sexual function problems and help seeking behaviour in Britain: national probability sample survey. *BMJ*, **327**, 426–427.

CHAPTER 7

Male Dermatoses

Manu Shah[1] and Chris Bunker[2]

[1]Burnley General Hospital, East Lancashire, UK
[2]Chelsea & Westminster and University College Hospitals, London, UK

OVERVIEW

- Rashes on the male genitalia may be part of a common dermatosis such as eczema or psoriasis or a disease specific to the genitals
- Taking an adequate history and performing a complete examination are crucial to making a diagnosis
- Genital dermatoses often have a profound effect on a man's relationships, libido and self-esteem
- Men are unlikely to discuss symptoms of genital rashes
- Most dermatoses can be easily treated and have a good outcome.

Diagnosing genital rashes

Patients presenting with rashes on the body such as eczema or psoriasis will not routinely ask about treatment for the same problem on the genitals.

Taking a good history will often give a diagnosis even before the genitals are examined. Symptoms may be non-specific and may be common to a number of dermatoses (Box 7.1). A sexual history (Chapter 5) and genital examination (Chapter 6) are necessary but particular attention must be directed to the symptoms of genital and general dermatoses as well as examining for specific signs, unique to genital skin problems. It is important to be aware of the wide variation of normality encountered eg pearly penile papules (Fig. 7.1)

Box 7.1 **Common symptoms of genital dermatoses**

- Red rash
- Itch
- Soreness especially with sex: *male dyspareunia*
- Scaly skin
- Penile discharge (from under the foreskin rather than the urethra)
- Difficulty retracting the foreskin

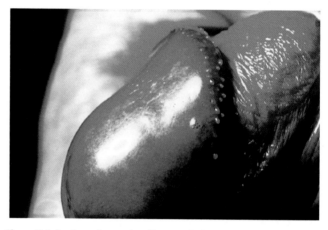

Figure 7.1 Pearly penile papules. (Courtesy Dr D.A. Burns, Leicester, UK)

Dermatoses of the genitals can be divided into those confined to the genitals and those that are part of a general inflammatory dermatosis (Box 7.2). However, many common inflammatory dermatoses such as eczema, lichen planus and psoriasis may only manifest on the genitals.

Box 7.2 **Classification of genital rashes**
Dermatoses confined to the genitals

- Zoon's balanitis (Figure. 7.2)
- Lichen sclerosus (Figure. 7.3)
- Pre-malignant lesions

Common inflammatory dermatoses with a genital manifestation

- Eczema
- Psoriasis
- Lichen planus (Figure. 7.4)

Genital problems in the absence of skin disease (dysmorphophobia; dysaesthesia)

Balanitis refers to inflammation of the glans and posthitis to inflammation of the foreskin. Most men with genital dermatoses are uncircumcised and present the differential

---

ABC of Sexual Health, Third Edition. Edited by Kevan Wylie.
© 2015 John Wiley & Sons, Ltd. Published 2015 by John Wiley & Sons, Ltd.

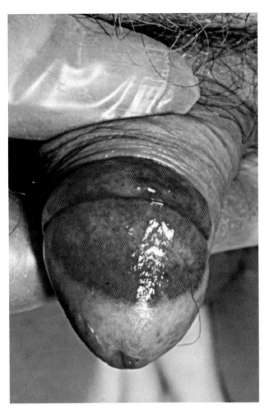

Figure 7.2 Zoon's balanitis. Asymptomatic, symmetrical moist erythema of glans and prepuce. (Courtesy of Professsor C.B. Bunker, with permissions from Medical Illustration, UK, Chelsea & Westminster Hospital, London, UK).

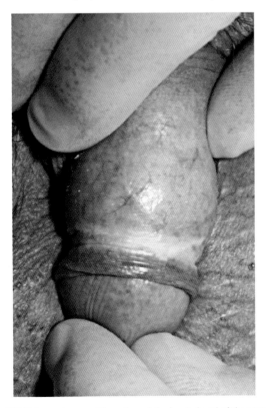

Figure 7.3 Lichen sclerosus. Circumferential sclerotic band of the prepuce causing 'waisting' and a constrictive posthitis. (Courtesy of Professsor C.B. Bunker, with permissions from Medical Illustration, UK, Chelsea & Westminster Hospital, London, UK).

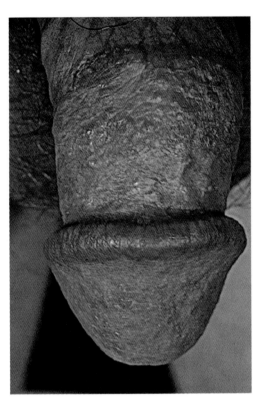

Figure 7.4 Lichen planus. Papules and annular lesions with Wickham's striae on the glans and shaft. (Courtesy of Professsor C.B. Bunker, with permissions from Medical Illustration, UK, Chelsea & Westminster Hospital, London, UK).

diagnosis of balanoposthitis. Most men who develop balanitis are uncircumcised and forms such as Zoon's balanitis and lichen sclerosus do not occur in circumcised men. However, balanitis of the circumcised penis may occur, for example due to eczema or psoriasis. Diabetes mellitus may need to be excluded.

Balanoposthitis presents with the symptoms of itching, soreness, penile discharge and tightness of the foreskin. There are a number of common causes (Box 7.3). Clinical features may vary according to the aetiology of the balanitis (Box 7.4).

Box 7.3 **Causes of balanitis and posthitis**

Inflammatory dermatosis (e.g. eczema, psoriasis, lichen sclerosus, lichen planus, Zoon's balanitis)

Infective balanoposthitis (e.g. candida, sexually transmitted infections, anaerobic bacteria)

Contact balanitis (e.g. irritant due to poor hygiene, excess use of detergents or allergic due to contact hypersensitivity, for example rubber or preservatives in medicaments or toiletries)

Lichen sclerosus (LSc)

LSc is an uncommon, chronic inflammatory dermatosis of uncircumcised men associated with scarring and a low incidence of squamous cell carcinoma. The true incidence is unknown. Although many still believe that it is an autoimmune disease all the evidence points to male genital LSc being due to chronic occluded

Box 7.4 Clinical features and management of balanitis

Type of balanitis	Clinical features	Management
Inflammatory dermatosis	See under eczema, psoriasis, lichen planus, lichen sclerosus	See under eczema, psoriasis, lichen planus
Infective balanoposthitis	Usually sore/burning glans	Exclude immunosuppression (e.g. diabetes)
	Redness/erosions of glans	Exclude STD
	Candida balanitis common in diabetes and obesity	Topical and/or oral treatment directed at the organism responsible
		Good hygiene
Contact balanoposthitis	Dry, glazed skin, eczematous in nature	Good hygiene
		Topical emollients
		Topical steroids
		Avoiding irritants, for example soap
Dermatoses confined to the genitals		
Zoon's balanoposthitis (Figure 7.2)	Elderly uncircumcised men, well demarcated moist red patches on glans with corresponding lesion(s) on foreskin	
	Staining of underwear with blood	
	Often asymptomatic	
	Is the diagnosis correct? Consider biopsy	Good hygiene
	Probably a form of chronic irritant mucositis	Topical steroids +/− anti-infective agents
		Circumcision

STD: sexually transmitted disease.

exposure of a susceptible epithelium to urine. Affected men 'dribble', that is, manifest terminal urinary microincontinence. LSc may present in a large variety of ways (Box 7.5 and Figure 7.3) with itching, soreness and problems with the foreskin (such as splitting, tightness and dyspareunia) being most common. Clinically, lesions usually appear on the penis as white or red patches and plaques, although a variety of clinical presentations may occur (Box 7.5). Left untreated, the condition often progresses to severe scarring.

Box 7.5 Clinical presentation of lichen sclerosus

Symptoms	Signs
• asymptomatic	• lichenoid or "Zoonoid" or mixed inflammation
• red/white patches	
• itch/burn/pain/blisters	• atrophic red/white (sclerotic) patches/plaques
• dyspareunia	
• tight foreskin	• telangiectasia/purpura
• difficulty with micturition	• erosions/ulceration
	• loss of architecture: narrow meatus, loss of frenulum, loss of pearly penile papules
• dysuria	
	• phimosis

The condition is usually diagnosed clinically but skin biopsy may occasionally be necessary if the clinical features are non-specific or if there is a suspicion of malignant change (e.g. if the lesion is verrucous, eroded or not responding to treatment). Both medical and surgical therapy may be necessary for patients. Active inflammatory disease may be treated under supervision with ultrapotent topical steroids. Soap substitution and the avoidance of contact with urine

and pubic hair is advised. A perimeatal barrier preparation is recommended. Failure to respond to medical treatment usually means the patient will require a circumcision. Close liaison with the urology team may be necessary as patients may require not just simple circumcision but frenuloplasty, meatotomy and meatal dilatation and complex plastic surgical repairs.

Pre-malignant lesions

Fixed red patches, plaques and papules on the penis may indicate pre-malignant lesions. It is important to consider this as a differential diagnosis in many inflammatory dermatoses of the genitals. Lesions may mimic a range of inflammatory problems such as Zoon's balanitis and one or more diagnostic biopsies may be necessary. The terminology is confusing with terms such as penile intraepithelial neoplasia, Erythroplasia of Queyrat, Bowenoid papulosis and Bowen's disease being used. However, all of these variants share a similar histological picture of carcinoma *in situ*.

Clinically, isolated lesions appear on the glans penis usually in uncircumcised men. However, erythema may be extensive, mimicking Zoon's and other forms of balanitis. Symptoms may be non-specific or absent. Symptoms include redness of the glans, itching, pain, bleeding, ulceration or isolated lesions. There should be a low level of suspicion when considering biopsy (see Box 7.6).

The management of pre-malignant lesions is specialized and patients should be seen by a local or regional specialist, skilled in treating such patients. Treatment options include surgery (including circumcision), topical 5-fluorouracil, laser ablation and photodynamic therapy.

Box 7.6 : **When to consider a diagnostic genital biopsy**

- asymmetric lesions
- isolated lesions
- unexplained ulceration or hyperkeratosis
- persistent lesions unresponsive to medical treatment
- diagnostic doubt

Common inflammatory dermatoses with a genital manifestation

Eczema

Eczema (dermatitis) is a common dermatosis and may be classified by aetiology into exogenous eczema (allergic contact dermatitis and irritant contact dermatitis) or endogenous (seborrhoeic eczema and atopic eczema) (Box 7.7). Lesions may be acute, chronic or acute-on-chronic. The predominant symptom is of itch. Rashes may be red, scaly and excoriated when acute or lichenified and pigmented when chronic. Problems may be exacerbated by secondary bacterial, fungal or yeast infection.

Box 7.7 **Symptoms and signs of eczema**

	Symptoms	Signs
Acute eczema (e.g. allergic contact dermatitis)	Pain, burning, itching	Erythema, localized swelling of skin, vesicles, exudation, paraphimosis
Chronic eczema (e.g. longstanding atopic eczema)	Chronic itch especially at night, burning, pain	Excoriations, lichenified skin, nodules (especially on scrotum), often evidence of eczema elsewhere on the body

Contact dermatitis on the genitals may be due to irritants such as soaps, shower gels, toiletries or products to enhance sex or allergens such as preservatives in topical agents (Box 7.8).

Seborrhoeic dermatitis is a papulo-squamous skin disorder usually localized to sebum-rich areas of the body including hairy areas. It may just be confined to the genitals but will usually also be seen on typical areas such as the scalp, naso-labial folds, eyebrows and eyelash areas. The condition is very common with a prevalence of 5% in healthy individuals but up to 85% in HIV-infected patients. The symptoms are of mild itching, tingling and even burning of the skin.

Redness, scaling and crusting are invariably present to some degree. The condition responds to topical steroid/anti-fungal combinations but relapse is common. The differential diagnosis includes psoriasis. The general management of genital eczema is detailed above (Box 7.9).

Psoriasis

Psoriasis affects at least 2% of the UK and US populations. Psoriasis on the genitals may be the only presentation of the disease.

Box 7.8 **Examples of contact allergens causing problems on the genitals**

Where allergen originates from	Source	Examples	Specific sensitizers
Direct contact	Medicaments and skin care products	Topical steroids, emollients, local anaesthetic creams, antibiotics, antifungals, bath products	Parabens, ethylene diamine, sorbic acid, propylene glycol and so on
	Contraceptives	Condoms	Latex, spermicides, rubber chemicals
Allergen transfer	Hands	Industrial allergens	Nickel, epoxies
	Partner	Feminine products	Fragrances

Typical irritants of the genital region

- Soaps, shower gels and other toiletries
- Urine, faeces
- Sweat, sebum
- Condoms, spermicides and products to enhance sex
- Sexual secretions
- Tight clothing and friction

Box 7.9 **Management of genital eczema**

- Identify any contact allergen or irritant
- Avoid contact allergens and irritants
- Use topical emollients
- Use soap substitutes
- Short-term use of topical steroids (+/− anti-infective agents)

The condition is often referred to as inverse psoriasis when intertriginous sites (e.g. axillae, natal cleft, groins and gluteal folds) are affected. The diagnosis may be difficult especially in the uncircumcised man. The skin lesions tend not to be scaly but are red and often smooth and shiny. The clinician needs to look for other signs of skin disease on the body (e.g. pits, onycholysis, oil drop lesions and hyperkeratosis in the nails) (Box 7.10). The diagnosis is usually made clinically but occasional tests such as skin biopsy may be necessary.

Some conventional treatments for psoriasis are contra-indicated on the genitals, for example phototherapy and crude tar preparations (risk of genital cancer). Others such as topical vitamin A and D analogues may be irritant in some patients. Topical therapy involves regular use of emollients and soap substitutes with

Box 7.10 **Typical sites for psoriasis**

- nails, scalp and ears
- umbilicus, sacrum, buttocks, natal cleft
- pubic mound, groins, penile shaft, glans and foreskin

Box 7.11 **Psoriasis management**

Diagnosis	Treatment
History including family history	Topical emollients
General examination especially scalp, nails and so on.	Short-term topical steroids
May be difficult in uncircumcised men	Avoid irritant products (e.g. deodorants, sexual enhancers)
1. Consider HIV infection in severe cases	
2. Skin biopsy may occasionally be needed	

General factors

- avoid friction (e.g. tight fitting underwear)
- use waterbased lubricants for sexual intercourse

Box 7.12 **Clinical features of lichen planus**

Symptoms	Sites commonly affected	Clinical features
Intense itch/burn	Palms and soles, wrists and ankles	Flat-topped purple/white shiny papules and plaques with lacy surface (Wickham's striae)
Dyspareunia	Mouth and genitals	May be discrete or confluent, Koebnerise
	Nails	Non-specific balanitis, discrete lesions, annular lesions on penis. Erosive disease

Box 7.13 **The following questions may aid a diagnosis of dysmorphophobia**

1 Are you worried about your appearance? What is your concern?
2 Does this concern preoccupy you? Do you think about it a lot and wish you could worry about it less?
3 What effect has this problem with your appearance had on your life? Has it caused you a lot of distress? Has it significantly interfered with your social life, family and friends, work or other aspects of your life?

intermittent use of topical steroids. Occasional topical antifungal, antiseptic or antibiotic therapy may be necessary. Severe genital psoriasis will respond to systemic agents such as biological agents, acitretin, methotrexate and ciclosporin. An overview of psoriasis management is detailed in Box 7.11.

Lichen planus

Lichen planus is a common inflammatory dermatosis that often affects the genitals in both men and women. The cause is unknown and the disease is usually self-limiting. Typically, the rash is symmetrical and itchy/burning. Classical sites may be involved (Box 7.12).

Lichen planus usually responds to topical steroids, although treatment may need to be prolonged. Erosive genital disease rarely responds to anything other than circumcision.

Dysmorphophobia and dysaesthesia

Dysmorphophobia, also known as body dysmorphic syndrome, describes patients with an imagined physical defect. The fixation may be on the genitals. Patients have a persistent belief of serious illness and will have repeated examinations and investigations. Some patients will undergo surgical treatments and enhancements to try to correct their so-called abnormality. The condition is

very difficult to manage and repeated reassurances rarely help. There is a strong association with other psychiatric illness such as suicidal ideation, depression and obsessive–compulsive disorder. Outcome seems to be poor but many authorities advocate a combination of psychotherapy and psychopharmacological treatments (Box 7.13).

Dysaesthesia syndromes manifest as inordinate dermatological symptomatology such as itching, burning, redness or pain in the absence of an identifiable dermatosis. Soap substitution, moisturization, topical moisturizers and oral antihistamines can be used. Topical steroids should be avoided. Low doses of dothiepin and dosulepin can help. Some patients respond to acupuncture.

Penile oedema

There are many causes of penile oedema (Box 7.14). There is no unifying classification currently. It is important to establish an underlying diagnosis so that therapy may be optimal. Some cases are labelled 'idiopathic' but such a label should only be used when other conditions have been excluded. Oedema of the penis may give rise to a number of problems including infection, urinary retention and sexual dysfunction.

Box 7.14 **Causes of penile oedema**

Cause	Examples
Malignancy and cancer treatment	Penile cancer, lymphoma, post-radiotherapy, post-lymph node dissection
Infection	Sexual, for example gonorrhoea Non-sexual, for example filariasis, cellulitis
Fluid overload	Heart failure with peripheral oedema
Congenital	Milroy's disease
Idiopathic	Chronic idiopathic penile oedema
Inflammatory	Hidradenitis, allergic contact dermatitis, Crohn's disease, sarcoidosis
Traumatic/post-operative	Implantation of penile filling devices, use of occlusive bands

The management of penile oedema is directed mainly at treating the underlying cause. There are some important general measures for all patients:

- Long term antibiotics are usually necessary
- Manual techniques to help lymphatic drainage
- Attention to skin hygiene
- Medical taping may be used in some patients
- Compression underwear may be helpful in some men
- Exercises devised by a lymphoedema therapist

Further reading

Bunker, C.B. (2004) *Male Genital Skin Disease.* Elsevier Saunders, reprinted 2005.

Bunker, C.B. & Neill, S.A. (2010) The genital, perianal and umbilical regions. In: Burns, T., Breathnach, S., Cox, N. & Griffiths, C. (eds), *Rook's Textbook of Dermatology,* 8th edn. Vol. **71**. Wiley-Blackwell, New York, pp. 1–102.

Shah, M. (2008) *The Male Genitalia: a Clinician's Guide to Skin Problems and Sexually Transmitted Infections.* Radcliffe, Oxford.

Veale, D., Eshkevari, E., Read, J., Miles, S., Troglia, A., Phillips, R., Echeverria, L.M., Fiorito, C., Wylie, K. & Muir, G. (2014) Beliefs about penis size: validation of a scale for men with shame about the size of their penis. *Journal of Sexual Medicine,* **11**, 84–92.

CHAPTER 8

Female Dermatoses

Ruth Murphy

Nottingham University Teaching Hospitals, Nottingham, UK

> **OVERVIEW**
>
> - Female genital dermatoses are common and are frequently incorrectly diagnosed as candida albicans
> - Simple care of the vulva, avoiding fragranced wash products and washing with emollients instead of soap will help most vulval dermatoses
> - Dermatoses may predominantly affects the vulval region such as lichen sclerosus
> - Common skin conditions may also affect the vulval region such as dermatitis and psoriasis
> - Common over-the-counter products such as local anaesthetic creams and feminine hygiene products may cause allergic contact dermatitis.

Common symptoms of vulval dermatoses

Inflammatory conditions which affect the vulval region are common. When a patient presents with vulval symptoms such as irritation or discomfort often the focus of the consultation is to exclude infection or malignancy and then reassure the patient. However, without a knowledge of inflammatory dermatoses such as lichen sclerosus or psoriasis, it is easy to underestimate the impact these conditions have on affected individuals and to deliver sub-optimal treatment.

The patient with an inflammatory vulval skin condition (dermatosis), usually presents with soreness, itch (pruitius vulvae) and/or discharge. Scratching in response to these symptoms, often sometimes at night, leads to lichenification, erosions and secondary infection (Figure 8.1). This results in significant discomfort, pain on passing urine, forced alterations in usual clothing and a challenge to sexual relationships.

Sadly, as these conditions are often chronic, years of unhappiness and eventual relationship breakdown are commonplace. However, most inflammatory dermatoses with accurate diagnosis can be easily treated and this alleviates unnecessary suffering.

Care of the vulva

The skin of the labia minora is thin and is easily irritated. Simple measures such as adopting a vulval hygiene and care strategy will bring almost instant relief and keep the skin in good condition. In short, this means avoiding common irritants such as soaps, perfumed shower gels and bubble baths and washing instead with a bland emollients such as hydramol. The application of any suitable emollient, such as Diprobase™ at night can also be applied and keep the skin in good condition.

What to be weary of with vulval disease

Patients presenting with vulval problems, before seeking medical advice, have often self-diagnosed and self-treated for 'thrush' or non-specific 'female irritation'. This is an important part of the history to elicit as these over-the-counter products may lead to an allergic contact dermatitis. This can actually *mask* any underlying vulval dermatosis. The fissures or excoriations in vulval skin conditions will often become secondarily infected with bacteria or yeast. It is only after these are treated that it will be possible to gain adequate control of any underlying vulval dermatoses.

In the next few paragraphs, the presentation and management of common vulval dermatoses will be discussed. These are largely divided into two groups, inflammatory skin conditions which predominantly affect the genital region such as lichen sclerosus and general skin conditions which can also affect the genital region such as psoriasis.

Pruritus vulvae

Pruritus vulvae is not a diagnosis. The term describes the symptoms of an itchy vulva attributable to many causes. The common skin problems which lead to an itchy vulva (pruritus vulvae) are lichen simplex chronicus, atopic vulvitis, vulval psoriasis, lichen sclerosus and lichen planus and many more. All these disorders may become complicated by infection with bacteria or yeast or contact dermatitis from the purchase of over-the-counter preparations.

Vulval pain

Many disorders affecting the vulva can lead to fissures and tears which become painful and lead to vulval pain. Again, this is not

ABC of Sexual Health, Third Edition. Edited by Kevan Wylie.
© 2015 John Wiley & Sons, Ltd. Published 2015 by John Wiley & Sons, Ltd.

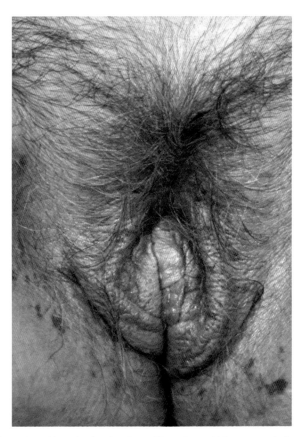

Figure 8.1 Lichen simplex chronicus with erosions which are secondarily infected

a diagnosis but is a symptom and, the underlying disorder requires correct diagnosis to provide adequate symptomatic relief. Vulvodynia is a diagnosis of exclusion and is diagnosed when there is no underlying cause for the vulval pain. It should be categorized as localized or generalized, provoked or unprovoked. This disorder is challenging to diagnose and manage. It usually requires secondary care input to control the symptoms.

Lichen simplex chronicus

This is a chronic irritating condition of the vulva which results in characteristic skin surface changes. Affected individuals are caught in an itch scratch cycle. The scratching temporarily relieves the irritation prompting more scratching which damages the overlying skin with subsequent lichenification. Examination of the vulval skin as in Figure 8.1 shows lichenified (thickened) skin with erosions. These erosions often become secondarily infected with staphylococcal, streptococcal or candida species.

The treatment is to break the itch scratch cycle and treat any underlying infection. To break the itch scratch cycle a potent topical steroid is usually required, applied at night for 2 weeks, with the liberal use of emollient during the day. It is then important to try and identify the cause of the triggering irritation. This could be from several sources but common causes to consider are irritant dermatitis from urinary incontinence or pads, iron deficiency anaemia or mild atopic vulvitis and psoriasis.

Lichen sclerosus

Lichen sclerosus is one of the commonest presentations of an intractably itchy vulva, particularly in post-menopausal women. In the early stages, it is frequently misdiagnosed as 'thrush'. The irritation caused by lichen sclerosus will often commence around the clitoris but may extend to the perianal region in a classical figure of eight distribution. The early symptoms are usually intractable itch, often worse at night, but as the disease progresses the affected skin will easily tear, particularly in the region of the posterior fourchette. This makes sexual activity painful and a common presenting symptom is tearing at the base of the introitus with sexual intercourse. On examination, the classical triad of poorly controlled active disease are pallor, atrophy and haemorrhage as seen in Figure 8.2.

Treatment with a reducing course of topical supra-potent topical steroids is excellent at gaining disease control (BAD guidelines, 2010). There are no head-to-head studies to indicate which treatment regimen is better. A regularly used regime is daily for 1 month followed by alternate days for 1 month then one to two times per week for the longer term.

Most individuals, when their lichen sclerosus is under control, wonder if therapy can be discontinued and will often cease to apply the steroid cream. In most instances though, the disease will re flare. In order to switch off the inflammatory process, it is necessary to repeat the treatment cycle. This is, applying the supra-potent topical steroids to the affected area in accordance with one of the published treatment regimens.

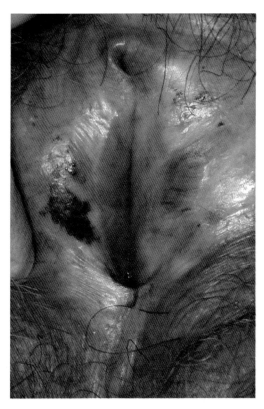

Figure 8.2 Lichen sclerosus affecting the vulva showing pallor, haemorrhage and tearing at the posterior fourchette

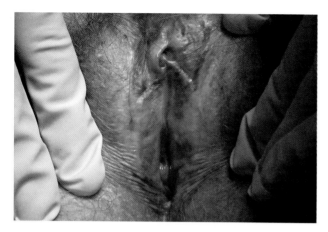

Figure 8.3 Lichen sclerosus at a later stage with post-inflammatory pigmentation loss of architecture and fissures in the labia minora

Individuals may worry about the thinning affects of topical steroids and need reassurance for their continued use. They may attribute the poor control of the lichen sclerosus to the side effects of the topical steroids and all this hinders compliance. This is easy to understand given that the vulval skin in undertreated lichen sclerosus will lead to thinning, tearing with fissures with loss of normal architecture (Figure 8.3). Many patients, misunderstanding the pathology of the disease, equate these changes as caused by the steroid creams rather than the inflammatory disorder.

Eventually, the vaginal introitus may become narrowed. Adhesions over the clitoris can result in a pseudocyst which can in turn become infected and painful. A small percentage of individuals (estimated at 5%) may be at risk of malignant transformation, with the development of a squamous cell carcinoma as shown in Figure 8.4. It is not known whether undertreatment of the condition increases the risk of malignant transformation, but certain forms of lichen sclerosus those with hypertrophic disease or on histological

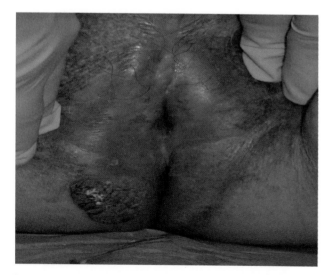

Figure 8.4 Advanced lichen sclerosus showing introital narrowing and burying of the clitoris. There is also a squamous cell carcinoma on the right buttock

reporting have differentiated vulval intraepithelial neoplasia are at increased risk.

Children also develop lichen sclerosus and appropriate use of supra-potent topical steroids needs to be particularly emphasized in this group, to preserve the normal vulval architecture and sexual function into adulthood. All affected children should really be under a specialist and the need for continued use of topical steroids requires frequently emphasizing during clinic visits.

Allergic and irritant contact dermatitis affecting the genital region

It is easy to forget that patients with vulval conditions will often buy over-the-counter creams and gels. Preparations such as topical anaesthetic creams for 'feminine itch' or fragranced products for 'feminine hygiene' and Canesten HC™ may sensitize susceptible individuals. A reaction to an allergen will peak at 48–96 h, making it difficult to 'work out' without patch-testing, the likely sensitizing agent. The presentation of contact dermatitis might be acute but often becomes chronic complicating a lichen simplex chronicus. Sometimes, it is a cyclical vulval irritation due to a sanitary pad which largely settles as menstruation is over only to re flare the following month. Figure 8.5 shows a contact dermatitis to a fragrances and bleaching agents in a sanitary pad. The use of a different pad, unbleached and fragrance free should be suggested.

Vulval psoriasis

Psoriasis is a very common inflammatory skin condition occurring in 1 in 50 of the population in the UK. The genital area is frequently affected in one of two ways, the natal cleft extending down to the anal margin, which usually fissures and frequently becomes secondarily infected and the hair-bearing skin of the labia majora as shown in Figure 8.6. When the mons pubis and the crural folds are affected, there are usually well demarcated erythematous plaques as shown in Figure 8.6. These are often less scaly than typical plaques of psoriasis and may present as vulval itch. It is usually very difficult

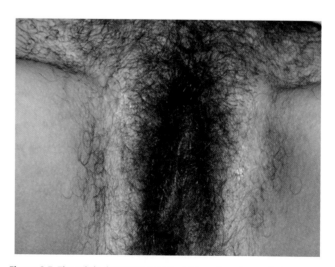

Figure 8.5 The subtle dermatitis over the labia majora demonstrates an allergic contact dermatitis affecting the vulva

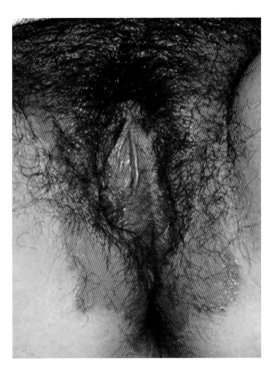

Figure 8.6 Psoriasis affecting the vulval region showing well demarcated erythematous plaques

to completely clear these plaques. However, treatment with emollients following the vulval care pathways can significantly relieve symptoms.

If the area becomes infected this requires treatment, otherwise pulsed therapy with topical steroids and calcineurin inhibitors is the mainstay of therapy. Sometimes, individuals only have psoriasis in the genital region, umbilicus and their scalp. It may not occur to them that the vulval problems are related to the skin lesions elsewhere. It is therefore necessary to ask patients with psoriasis if they have any genital discomfort or irritation so as not to miss an opportunity to treat.

Atopic vulvitis

Vulval eczema as part of atopic eczema is particularly common in young children. Like patients with psoriasis, it is easy for patients not to think that their eczema can affect the vulval region. This condition is very easily relieved using vulval hygiene and emollient strategies. Any secondary infection needs treating and the inflammation controlled with pulsed topical steroids of appropriate potency for the grade of atopic vulvitis.

Conclusion

Inflammatory skin diseases commonly occur on the vulva. They can be relieved with simple vulval care, avoiding soaps and using emollients. Correct diagnosis is required however to provide maximum disease control.

Further reading

BAD (0000) The British Association of Dermatologists Patient Information Leaflet for;Care of vulval skin/Lichen sclerosus/ Vulvodynia, http://www.bad.org.uk/ (accessed 4 December 2014).

Neill, S.M., Lewis, F.M., Tatnall, F.M., Cox, N.H. & British Association of Dermatologists (2010) British Association of Dermatologists' guidelines for the management of lichen sclerosus. *British Journal of Dermatology*, **163** (**4**), 672–682.

The British Society for the Study of Vulvo vaginal Disease (0000) http://www.bssvd.org/ (accessed 4 December 2014).

CHAPTER 9

Investigation and Management of Endocrine Disorders Affecting Sexuality

T. Hugh Jones[1,2]

[1]Barnsley Hospital NHS Foundation Trust, Barnsley, UK
[2]University of Sheffield, Sheffield, UK

OVERVIEW

- Fatigue is a common symptom in any endocrine disease which may affect sexual as well as general health
- To make a diagnosis of male hypogonadism, symptoms as well as biochemical evidence of testosterone deficiency must be present
- The three sexual symptoms associated with hypogonadism are loss or reduced libido, loss or reduced morning erections and erectile dysfunction
- Testosterone replacement therapy must be monitored regularly by a trained medical practitioner
- HRT is the treatment of choice in premature ovarian failure, but low-dose testosterone may improve libido if this symptom persists.

Introduction

Any endocrine disorder which causes hormonal imbalance adversely affects wellbeing and quality of life which does compromise sexual as well as general health. Testosterone and oestrogens have specific and essential roles in sexual health, but deficiency of each of these hormones does also affect physical, mental and general health.

Testosterone in men

Physiology

Testosterone is produced and secreted but not stored by the testes. The release of testosterone is controlled by the pulsatile release of gonadotrophin-releasing hormone (GnRH) from the hypothalamus which then stimulates release of luteinizing hormone (LH) from the pituitary. LH then directly stimulates testosterone synthesis and release with testosterone having a negative feedback on the hypothalamic–pituitary axis to maintain a balance in testosterone levels in the blood. There is a circadian rhythm of testosterone release with levels highest between 0600 and 0800 hours and then falling to a nadir between 1800 and 2000 hours. The reason for this

rhythm is unknown, but is important to recognize that blood for testosterone measurement should be taken before 1100 hours to standardize assessment for diagnosis of testosterone deficiency.

Circulating testosterone is made of three different fractions: free (2–3%), albumen-bound (20–50%) and sex hormone binding globulin (SHBG)-bound (Figure 9.1). The free and albumen-bound testosterone is biologically active, whereas SHBG-bound testosterone is considered to be inactive as the testosterone is tightly bound to this carrier protein.

The major biological actions of testosterone are to promote the development of secondary sexual characteristics, develop and maintain sexual health as well as many important effects on general and physical health. Apart from the well-known effects on muscle strength and bulk, testosterone is essential for bone health, reducing body fat composition, cognitive function, cardiovascular health and carbohydrate and fat metabolism.

Hypogonadism (sometimes known as testosterone deficiency syndrome – TDS) is a clinical syndrome complex which comprises both symptoms (with or without clinical signs) and biochemical evidence of testosterone deficiency.

Symptoms and signs

The three most common symptoms of hypogonadism are related to sexual health and consist of reduced or loss of libido and morning/nocturnal erections and erectile dysfunction. Other common symptoms include fatigue and lethargy, reduce physical strength and endurance, loss of vitality, excessive sweating and psychological symptoms such as mood disturbance, grumpiness, irritability and a

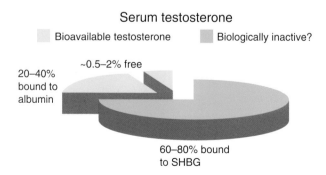

Figure 9.1 Serum testosterone

ABC of Sexual Health, Third Edition. Edited by Kevan Wylie.
© 2015 John Wiley & Sons, Ltd. Published 2015 by John Wiley & Sons, Ltd.

Table 9.1 Symptoms and signs of testosterone deficiency

Reduced/loss of libido
Reduced morning erections
Erectile dysfunction
Fatigue
Decreased muscle bulk and strength
Diminished physical or work performance
Decreased vitality
Loss of height
Hot flushes/sweats
Sleep disturbance
Lack of concentration and memory
Moodiness, grumpy, irritable
Reduced motivation/self-confidence
Feeling sad or blue/depressed mood
Infertility
Breast discomfort/gynaecomastia
Low trauma fracture/decreased bone mineral density
Increased percentage body fat
Loss of secondary sexual characteristics
Reduced shaving frequency
Small testes

Table 9.2 Common causes of hypogonadism

Primary testicular failure

Klinefelter's syndrome (XXY) 1 in 500 male births
Cryptorchidism – failure of testicular descent
Orchitis, for example mumps
Alcohol
HIV
Trauma/torsion of testes
Idiopathic (unknown)

Secondary (hypothalamic/pituitary) failure
Pituitary tumour (adenoma)
Hyperprolactinaemia (prolactinoma, drugs, hypothyroidism, pituitary stalk compression)
Parasellar brain tumour or metastases
Head injury
Systemic illness, for example type 2 diabetes
Haemochromatosis (iron storage disorder)
Chronic opiate analgesia or abuse
Chronic glucocorticoid treatment
Androgen deprivation therapy for prostate cancer
Congenital GnRH deficiency, for example Kallmann's syndrome

Late-onset hypogonadism
Testosterone deficiency after exclusion of classical causes of hypogonadism (see above)

Table 9.3 Investigations for hypogonadism

Screening in the presence of hypogonadal symptoms
Total testosterone (TT) before 1100 h
If TT <12 nmol/l repeat second TT with
LH, FSH
Prolactin
SHBG
If LH, FSH low or prolactin elevated investigate for structural pituitary lesion
MRI Pituitary
Check Ferritin
If LH FSH elevated Karyotype

tendency towards depression (Table 9.1). Hypogonadism may also be associated with delayed or failure of puberty, subfertility and gynaecomastia.

Signs of hypogonadism are usually only evident in men with very low testosterone. If the gonadal failure has occurred before puberty, they usually have a eunuchoid body shape, gynaecomastia, boyish face and lack of secondary sexual characteristics. Post-pubertal onset of hypogonadism may be associated with fine wrinkling of facial skin especially around the mouth.

Causes of hypogonadism

Primary hypogonadism is due to failure of testicular function and can be identified by elevated serum LH and follicle stimulating hormone (FSH) levels. The commonest classical cause is Klinefelter's syndrome in which the chromosome complement is usually XXY (Table 9.2).

Secondary hypogonadism (sometimes known as hypogonadotrophic hypogonadism) is caused by hypothalamic or pituitary failure with low or low normal LH and FSH. This condition may be caused by a pituitary tumour or other diseases which affects these structures. Secondary hypogonadism may also occur in relation to obesity, chronic opiate or glucocorticoid therapy where LH levels are inappropriately low in the setting of low testosterone. Significant hyperprolactinaemia (confirmed by measuring prolactin at least 30 minutes after cannualtion to exclude the effect of stress) suppresses GnRH release from the hypothalamus leading to low LH and FSF and as a result low testosterone. This is a form of secondary hypogonadism. The commonest causes of hyperprolactinaemia include a microprolactinoma (<1 cm diameter), compression of the pituitary stalk by pituitary adenomas or other tumours and primary hypothyroidism and commonly used drugs which include metoclopramide, sulpiride and tricyclic antidepressants). However no cause may be identified and this is known as idiopathic hyperprolactinaemia. Late-onset hypogonadism is associated with advancing age and characterised by symptoms and a deficiency in

serum testosterone levels when all classical causes of hypogonadsim have been excluded.

Investigations

Morning total testosterone must be measured on at least two occasions at least 1 week apart and sometimes more to confirm that the low testosterone state is persistent. For example, levels may be low in the presence of viral infection. If the initial sample is low, then LH, FSH and SHBG should be assessed along with sample 2 (Table 9.3). In borderline cases free testosterone should be calculated using Vermeulen's formula (www.issam.ch/freetesto.htm) using the following values total testosterone, SHBG and albumen. Prolactin and ferritin (haemochromatosis) should be measured if LH is low or low normal.

The cut-off values of total testosterone vary according to laboratory and assay used. However as the majority of normal ranges at the lower end have total testosterone levels around 8 nmol/l, then guidelines have used this figure below which hypogonadism can be diagnosed in the presence of symptoms. It is also recognized that symptomatic men with levels at the low end of normal may have hypogonadism. Guidelines recommend different cut-off values, for example 10.4 and 12 nmol/l. The diagnosis of hypogonadism can be substantiated by calculation of free testosterone <225 pmol/l.

The underlying cause of hypogonadism should be diagnosed if possible and importantly structural disorders of the hypothalamus and pituitary by MRI (magnetic resonance imaging) scanning. If hypopituitarism is suspected, then all pituitary hormones should be measured: ferritin if haemochromatosis suspected, prolactin in low LH and karyotype if Klinefelter's considered.

PSA and a digital rectal examination in men >40 years to exclude occult prostate carcinoma and full blood count (FBC) in all subjects should be done before initiation of testosterone replacement therapy (TRT).

Low testosterone is a biomarker for diabetes and/or cardiovascular disease. Men with hypogonadism should be fully assessed clinically for cardiovascular risk factors. In particular all should have a fasting glucose and if elevated an oral glucose tolerance test and a fasting lipid profile.

Management

Once hypogonadism has been diagnosed, prostate carcinoma should be excluded and the absence of any contraindications to TRT (see national and international guidelines) patients can be considered for a trial of therapy. The commonest formulations of testosterone used are the gels. Gels are presented in sachets, tubes or metered pumps. A dose of testosterone 50/60 mg per day should be commenced, then testosterone levels are checked in 3 weeks (2–4 hours post gel application); to be sure levels are in the mid-normal range usually >15 nmol/l. A dose titration may be necessary. There is also a testosterone solution applied to the axilla which is available in the USA. Testosterone undeconoate can be given as an intramuscular injection every 10–14 weeks after initial loading injections at 0 and 6 weeks. The frequency of injection can be altered to achieve trough testosterone levels to be maintained within the normal range. Other formulations include short-acting testosterone ester intramuscular injections, muco-adhesive buccal tablets, skin patches (in some countries), intra-abdominal pellets and oral tablets of which apart from buccal tablets and skin patches it is difficult to achieve steady-state mid-normal range testosterone levels.

Patients should be assessed after 3, 6 and 12 months to be sure that there has been a symptomatic improvement and no side-effects. If there has been no benefit, cessation of treatment should be considered.

Once established on treatment after 12 months, subjects should be reviewed on an annual basis by a trained professional. Dose titration may still be needed especially if weight loss has occurred. PSA and FBC should also be monitored at the subsequent annual visits. Hyperprolactinaemia should be treated with dopamine agonist drugs (cabergoline, bromocriptine or quinagolide). If the testosterone level does not normalise then testosterone supplementation may be necessary as a pituitary adenoma may have caused failure of the gonadotrophs to produce the gonadotrophins.

Testosterone in women

Testosterone is synthesized and secreted by the ovaries and the adrenal glands. The circulating levels of testosterone in women are approximately 10-fold lower than those in men. The ovaries also release dehydroepiandrostenedione (DHEA) and androstenedione, both precursors of testosterone.

The measurement of testosterone at these low levels does lead to problems in accuracy of the assays and therefore if testosterone replacement is given does not allow accurate replacement of testosterone to the normal range. This is further compounded by the fact that SHBG can fluctuate being raised by oestrogen, age and hyperthyroidism and lowered by obesity and hypothyroidism. Androgen status in women can be estimated by using the free androgen index (total testosterone/SHBG × 100).

There is a gradual decline in adrenal production of testosterone and its precursors with ageing. However, ovarian production is usually maintained after the menopause although there is a fall in DHEA and androstenedione. Clinical conditions which result in significantly decreased testosterone levels include bilateral oophorectomy, premature ovarian failure and hypopituitarism.

Low testosterone levels in women may have an adverse effect on libido, however this is by no means definite as some studies have not confirmed this. In a study of women with premature ovarian failure, women in whom the testosterone levels were highest did have an increased frequency of desire for sexual contact.

TRT in women is controversial and has only been licensed for use in women who have had bilateral oophorectomy. Placebo-controlled studies have reported mixed results with some showing an increase in sexual desire and others not. The studies have been short-term and mainly used testosterone patches or transdermal gels. However, the long-term safety of these therapies is unknown. In the short-term, the main side-effects as can be expected are acne and hirsutism. The Endocrine Society Task Force have advised against the use of testosterone and other androgens in women due to the lack of clear indications for treatment and no long-term safety studies.

Oestrogens

Ovarian failure may occur prematurely or naturally during the menopause. The symptoms of ovarian failure are well known and include fatigue, hot flashes, sweats, dyspareunia (due to reduced vaginal secretions) and changes in mood. Premature ovarian failure may be due to primary ovarian disorder (POF) which may occur, for example as a result of autoimmune disease or the causes may not be identified. This condition is confirmed by marked elevation in LH and FSH levels and low 17β-oestradiol. A small number of subjects with POF (approximately 5%) may recover spontaneously. Pituitary failure from a number of disorders may also lead to decreased gonadotrophin release (LH and FSH) causing secondary ovarian failure. Treatment of the underlying pituitary condition may lead to recovery of ovarian function. In the presence of primary ovarian failure or unresolved pituitary disease, the only potential treatment is that of hormone replacement therapy (HRT) with exogenous oestrogens (with or without progestins). In the presence of long-standing amenorrhoea (>12 months), then it is

Table 9.4 HRT for women risks versus benefits

Risks	Benefits
Thrombo-embolism	Suppresses hot flushes/sweats
Increased risk of stroke	Improves sexual function by increasing vaginal lubrication
Increased risk of breast cancer	Improves osteoporosis risk
Increased risk of endometrial and ovarian cancer	May improve urinary incontinence and reduce UTIs
Migraine?	May reduce risk of CVD
Gallstones	may improve mood, wellbeing QOL

advisable to commence therapy with low-dose estrogens gradually increasing the full replacement dose.

The menopause is responsible for sexual dysfunction in 40% of women. The main symptom is vaginal dryness causing dyspareunia as in POF. Libido may be reduced as a result of concomitant reductions in androgen production. In common with POF, the menopausal symptoms include sweats, hot flashes, mood changes (irritability, forgetfulness, reduced concentration and anxiety) and an increased risk of urinary tract infections. HRT if considered has to be weighed up with benefits versus risks (Table 9.4). Benefits include control of vasomotor symptoms, urinary and vaginal symptoms and protection against osteoporosis. Against this, HRT increases risks for venous thromboembolism, stroke, breast, endometrial and ovarian cancer, migraine and gallstones. A decision to treat should be made between the doctor and the patient based on the full knowledge of these facts.

Thyroid disorders

There is a higher prevalence of female sexual dysfunction in the presence of hypothyroidism, Hashimoto's thyroiditis and nodular goitre. A recent study reported a prevalence of 46.1% compared to 20.7% in controls. Specifically, the symptoms consisted of reduced desire, arousal and lubrication. Symptoms were more likely to be present with higher TSH levels.

In men, diminished erectile function may occur in hyperthyroidism and hypothyroidism.

Fatigue experienced in untreated hyperthyroidism or hypothyroidism could potentially contribute to reduced libido.

Adequate treatment of these conditions overtime may improve sexual function.

Diabetes

Females with diabetes either type 1 (27%) or type 2 (53%) have an increased prevalence of sexual dysfunction compared to the normal healthy population. They have reduced libido, arousal, lubrication, orgasm and overall sexual satisfaction. The symptoms worsen with duration of diabetes and age.

Up to 70% of men with diabetes have reported to have erectile dysfunction which may be multi-factorial including vasculopathy, neuropathy, hypogonadism, drug-related, abdominal obesity and psychological factors. The hypogonadism if present invariably contributes to the sexual dysfunction. Failure of phosphodiesterase inhibitor type 5 therapy may be due to low testosterone. TRT has been shown to improve the response to sildenafil in approximately 60% of men who previously failed to respond to this drug.

Conclusion

It is important to evaluate both men and women for endocrine disorders who present with sexual dysfunction as this could identify a treatable disorder.

Further reading

Bhasin, S., Cunningham, G.R. & Hayes, F.J. (2010) Testosterone therapy in men with androgen deficiency syndrome; an Endocrine Society clinical practise guideline. *The Journal of Clinical Endocrinology and Metabolism*, **95**, 1995–2010.

Jones, T.H. (2013) *Testosterone Deficiency in Men*, 2nd edn. Oxford University Press.

Nieschlag, E. & Behre, H.M. (eds) (2004) *Testosterone Action, Deficiency, Substitution*, 4th edn. Cambridge University Press, Cambridge.

Wang, C., Nieschlag, E. & Swerdloff, R. (2008) Investigation, treatment and monitoring of late-onset hypogonadism. *European Journal of Endocrinology*, **159**, 507–14.

Wylie, K., Rees, M., Hackett, G. *et al.* (2010) Androgens , health and sexuality in men and women. *Maturitas*, **67** (**3**), 275–289.

CHAPTER 10

Investigations in Sexual Medicine for Women and Men with Sexual Health Problems

Irwin Goldstein[1] and Kevan Wylie[2,3,4]

[1] Alvarado Hospital, CA, USA
[2] Sexual Medicine, Porterbrook Clinic and Urology, Sheffield, UK
[3] Honorary Professor of Sexual Medicine, University of Sheffield, UK
[4] World Association for Sexual Health

> ## OVERVIEW
> - A careful and systematic physical examination is necessary when managing certain sexual dysfunctions
> - For some conditions, biochemical and endocrinological profiles can assist in the diagnostic process
> - For some men and women, specialist investigations can provide valuable information in the differentiation of the aetiology for the dysfunction

The diagnostic investigations and treatment opportunities for women with sexual health concerns are limited, in large part, due to the lack of current global government-approved agents for any sexual health concerns (desire, arousal, orgasmic and sexual pain-related dysfunctions) of pre-menopausal women or for non-sexual pain concerns of post-menopausal women. There are, in contrast, more than 20 US government-approved treatment strategies for men with bothersome male sexual dysfunctions. The availability of safe and effective medicaments for men with sexual health problems has, in part, motivated clinicians to better understand the nature of men's sexual health concerns. This has led to more clinical diagnostic procedures for men with sexual dysfunction.

This chapter will focus on providing a detailed overview on the physical examination and investigations utilized to help diagnose women and men with bothersome sexual health complaints. The reader is referred to subsequent principal chapters for a detailed description of individual sexual problems and the contemporary management.

Problems of sexual desire, libido and arousal in women

Investigations for women with problems of sexual desire

Sexual excitation and sexual inhibition imbalance resulting in problems of sexual desire may be influenced by multiple factors (see Chapter 15).

The Decreased Sexual Desire Screener (DSDS) is a self-report questionnaire validated for hypoactive sexual desire disorder (HSDD) with four yes/no questions to establish the presence of an acquired, distressing, decrease in sexual desire that the patient would like to increase. The fifth question presents a number of potential causes or exacerbating factors for loss of desire. Patients who do not endorse all of the first four questions are unlikely to have HSDD as defined in DSM-IV.

Clinical assessment is also needed. Evaluation of problems of sexual desire should include a focused physical examination, including a pelvic examination, and if needed, vulvoscopy, especially if the health care provider suspects local genital pathology contributing to the sexual dysfunction.

Evaluation should start with careful inspection of the external genitalia including mons pubis, labia majora, labia minora, clitoris and vulvar vestibule. This initial examination may reveal genital lesions, erythema that may predispose to sexual pain disorders, redundancy of the labia or atrophy of the external genitalia which is common after menopause and in some women taking hormonal contraceptives.

Vulvoscopy with photography involves examination of external female genitalia using a binocular vulvoscope/colposcope with 4x, 6x, 10x, 16x and 25x magnification and light source. Vulvoscopic photographs document the health of various organs. For example, one can visualize the glans clitoris, the minor vestibular glands, the hymenal tissue, the labia minora and labia majora, the frenulae, the peri-urethral tissue, the vaginal mucosa and the cervix.

Laboratory testing may include measurements of testosterone, sex hormone binding globulin (SHBG), free testosterone, oestradiol, progesterone, luteinizing hormone (LH), follicle-stimulating hormone (FSH), prolactin and thyroid-stimulating hormone (TSH).

Testosterone is a sex steroid hormone that is naturally synthesized by the ovaries and the adrenal gland and numerous other tissues and has multiple physiological actions in women. Approximately 50% of circulating androgens in healthy women are derived from the adrenal glands with the remaining 50% derived from the ovaries. The level of free testosterone is influenced by binding of the hormone to SHBG and, in part, weaker binding, to albumin. Testosterone bound to SHBG tends not to exert biological effects.

ABC of Sexual Health, Third Edition. Edited by Kevan Wylie.
© 2015 John Wiley & Sons, Ltd. Published 2015 by John Wiley & Sons, Ltd.

Androgen receptors have been localized to female genital tissues. Testosterone plays important roles for women, including sexual appetitive behaviour, maintenance of genital tissue integrity and sexual arousal responses. Low androgen levels have been associated with declines in sexual activity and desire. Testosterone levels decline in women with age although the rate of decrease slows after age 35.

There is an association between hormone-based contraception and HSDD, due in part to the effect of decreased testosterone production and increased SHBG decreasing free testosterone levels. Hormone-based contraception-increased SHBG may persist years after termination of hormonal contraception. Oestrogen deficiency has been linked to vulvovaginal mucosal changes and dyspareunia that may secondarily contribute to HSDD.

Investigations for women with problems of sexual arousal

The clinical diagnosis of Female Sexual Arousal Disorder (FSAD) requires a biopsychosocial evaluation beginning with a clinical interview concerning the lack of subjective arousal and/or lack of genital arousal, adequacies of sexual stimuli and any predisposing factors (see Chapter 15).

Validated self-report measures such as the Female Sexual Function Index (FSFI) – arousal domain may be used.

Laboratory investigations such as measurements of testosterone, SHBG, free testosterone oestradiol, progesterone, LH, FSH, prolactin and TSH may be obtained.

A focused genital/pelvic examination, vulvoscopy, is indicated in FSAD especially when there are complaints of loss of genital sensitivity or lack of vaginal swelling or lubrication.

An evaluation should be made of the level of voluntary control of the pelvic floor muscles, pelvic floor muscle tonus, presence of vaginal wall prolapse, signs of vaginal atrophy, size of introitus, presence of discharge, or evidence of infection (acute or chronic), epithelial disorders and/or pain. Vaginal pH (acidity; normal </4.5), vaginal wet mount and smear should be obtained.

Additional specialist diagnostic laboratory studies that are helpful in certain circumstances include duplex Doppler ultrasonography, thermal imaging using forward looking infrared, magnetic resonance imaging of the pelvic area and vaginal photoplethysmography and thermal clearance.

Objective sensory nerve testing may be performed using a biothesiometer to determine vibratory perception thresholds, expressed in volts. Objective sensory nerve testing may be also performed using temperature testing to determine hot and cold perception threshold values, expressed in degrees centigrade using, for example the GSA. Quantitative sensory testing measures and values are obtained in a non-genital reference site (pulp index finger) as well as in multiple genital sites such as the glans clitoris (dorsal nerve branches of the pudendal nerve), and the right and left labia minora (the perineal nerve branches of the pudendal nerve). More research needs to be performed on the value of these studies in FSAD.

Persistent genital arousal disorder (PGAD)

Persistent genital arousal disorder (PGAD) is associated with unrelenting, unwanted, persistent, intrusive and spontaneous sensations such as pressure/discomfort, engorgement, pulsating, pounding and/or throbbing in the genital tissues such as the clitoris, labia, vagina and/or in the perineum and/or anus in the absence of conscious thoughts of sexual desire or sexual interest.

PGAD is often associated with significant personal bother and distress. Women with PGAD are often ashamed for having feelings in their genitals. Women with PGAD often have suicidal thoughts.

PGAD may be classified as primary, lifelong if the PGAD is present throughout the person's life or as secondary, acquired if the PGAD develops variably in later life. PGAD is associated with spontaneous orgasms or feelings that orgasm is imminent or feelings that orgasmic release is needed to reduce the feelings of persistent arousal, but where symptoms are not consistently diminished by orgasmic release. The prevalence of PGAD is unknown.

PGAD may be associated with psychological-related pathophysiologies. Women with PGAD have described that stress worsens PGAD symptoms, whereas distraction and relaxation strategies lessen PGAD symptoms.

PGAD may be associated with biological-related pathophysiologies including vascular, neurological, pharmacological, and hormonal aetiologies. Arterial vascular causes may be secondary to pelvic arterio-venous malformations with unregulated arterial communications to the genitalia. Venous vascular causes may be secondary to pelvic congestion syndrome with ovarian venous incompetence and large varices draining the genitalia.

Central neurological causes such as Tourette's syndrome, epilepsy, post-blunt central nervous system (CNS) trauma, post-neurosurgical intervention of central arterio-venous malformation, Tarlov cysts, or to cervical and lumbosacral surgical interventions have been associated with PGAD. Peripheral neurological causes may be secondary to pudendal nerve entrapment, hypersensitivity or small fibre neuropathy of the pudendal nerve including its dorsal branch to the clitoris.

Pharmacological causes include the use of certain antidepressants, such as trazodone or secondary to sudden withdrawal of selective serotonin reuptake inhibitors (SSRIs) as occurs in sudden SSRI discontinuation syndrome.

Hormonal causes may be secondary to initiation and discontinuation of hormone therapy in post-menopausal women.

Investigations in PGAD

Women with PGAD should undergo detailed history, psychological evaluation, physical examination and laboratory testing. Physical examination may be used to identify potential peripheral neurological causes secondary to pudendal nerve entrapment.

Hormone blood tests can be used to assess if hormonal causes or initiation and discontinuation of hormone therapy in post-menopausal women are associated with PGAD.

Clitoral ultrasound studies can be used to diagnose arterial vascular causes secondary to pelvic arterio-venous malformations with unregulated arterial communications to the genitalia. Pelvic ultrasound and transvaginal ultrasound can be used to exclude venous vascular causes secondary to pelvic congestion syndrome with ovarian venous incompetence and large varices draining the genitalia.

Neurological consultation, electroencephalogram (EEG), Computerized tomography (CT) scans, and magnetic resonance imagings (MRIs) may be utilized to diagnose central neurological causes from Tourette's syndrome, epilepsy, post-blunt CNS trauma, Tarlov cysts, post-neurosurgical intervention of central arterio-venous malformation or to cervical and lumbosacral surgical interventions.

Psychological-based treatments engage management of the depression or focus on efforts to maximize relaxation through strategies such as distraction and/or hypnosis.

Investigations for women with problems of orgasmic disorder

The clinical diagnosis of female orgasm disorder (FOD) is established by a biopsychosocial evaluation (see Chapter 18). Physiological approaches to improving orgasmic function focus on ruling out contributing medical causes. Similar physical examination, hormone, neurological and blood flow testing, as described for women with sexual arousal disorder, should be considered for women with orgasmic disorders.

Specifically, blood testing should be considered for sex hormone levels such as testosterone, SHBG, free testosterone, LH, FSH, oestradiol, progesterone, prolactin and TSH. These blood tests will assess ovarian function, pituitary function and thyroid function. If neuropathy is suspected, measure the full blood count (FBC), B12 and folate and glucose levels.

Investigations for women with problems of dyspareunia

A detailed clinical history is required (see Chapter 19) before considering a physical examination with vulvoscopy for women with dyspareunia. Vulvar skin conditions are common and can lead to a variety of sexual concerns, particularly sexual pain. Examples include generalized dermatological conditions such as eczema, psoriasis, contact dermatitis, fungal infections, aphthosis ulcers and drug reactions. Some dermatoses are specific to the vulva and include lichen simplex, lichen sclerosis and lichen planus (see Chapter 8).

After external evaluation is complete, examination of the internal genitalia and vagina should be performed. The examination should include bimanual examination to assess for pelvic organ prolapse and ovarian pathology, a potential cause of pain during intercourse.

Assessment of the levator ani should be included as part of the bimanual examination; assessment of pelvic floor muscle laxity or hypertonicity as well as point tenderness may be relevant in the work up of sexual pain disorders. Consideration should be given to performing a speculum examination to rule out cervical pathology.

Assessment of vaginal pH is a simple, inexpensive test. High pH implies oestrogen deficiency and/or disruption of the normal vaginal microbiome; this may have relevance to issues of recurrent infection, vulvovaginal atrophy, or other issues and should be considered as a routine given its minimal invasiveness and safety.

Specialist investigations may include skin biopsies if dermatoses or dysplasia, ultrasonography (vaginal, abdominal) and X-Ray (XR) or MRI of the lower back and/or pelvis.

Investigations for men with problems of sexual desire

After a careful clinical history (see Chapter 14), exclude affective disorders with use of a questionnaire such as the hospital anxiety and depression scale (HAD) (cut-off point of 8/21 for anxiety or depression). A clinical examination is usually recommended especially if indicated by co-morbid conditions.

Exclude hormonal disturbance – principally androgen and thyroid deficiency and hyperprolactinaemia (all non-fasting samples). If there is suspicion of low testosterone levels, it is worth administering the androgen deficiency in aging males (ADAM) questionnaire. A positive response to item 1 or 7 or to any other three items is compatible with (but not necessarily diagnostic of) hypogonadism.

Investigations for men with problems of erectile dysfunction

A detailed clinical history should be taken (see Chapter 16) before proceeding with a physical examination. The focused genital physical examination should be carried out in each patient presenting with erectile dysfunction. The following examinations should be considered: general appearance and secondary sexual characteristics of an individual with hypogonadism; a cardiovascular examination including blood pressure and peripheral pulses; a genital examination including inspection of the prepuce and glans, size and consistency of the testicles, size and shape of the penis and fibrotic plaques in the stretched penis consistent with Peyronie's disease; a digital rectal examination in patients over 40 years to evaluate the prostate size, shape, consistency and presence of masses; neurological examination for perineal and penile sensitivity; and assessment of anal sphincter tone and bulbocavernosus reflex where compression of the glans triggers anal contraction, as palpated during rectal examination.

The physician must tailor the laboratory work-up based on the patient's complaints and risk factor exposure such as diabetes (obtain blood glucose and haemoglobin $A1_C$), hyperlipidaemia (obtain lipid profile and endothelial function blood tests), hypertension (obtain blood pressure and pulse, serum creatinine and blood urea nitrogen (BUN)) or coronary artery disease (obtain electrocardiogram (ECG)).

Total testosterone and free testosterone should also be measured in the morning in men under age 50 years, especially with erectile dysfunction and low libido. Diurinal variation of testosterone is less pronounced in men over age 50, so their testosterone blood tests can be performed even in the afternoon. Since SHBG increases with increasing age, and since SHBG tightly binds to testosterone and thus decreases bioavailable or free unbound testosterone, the more reliable measure of the presence of hypogonadism is the measurement of free androgen index defined by the ratio of total testosterone to SHBG. Assays for total testosterone particularly in the middle-aged men may not reflect the man's true androgenic status. SHBG decreases with obesity and conditions such as hypothyroidism and diabetes mellitus.

Other endocrine blood tests that may be useful to diagnose the endocrine milieu include LH, FSH and prolactin. Also TSH may identify an unsuspected hypothyroid state. Oestradiol determination may be relevant in men with elevated body mass indexes as there is high aromatase activity in men with excess adipose tissue. Dihydrotestosterone may be useful to diagnose the integrity of the 5-alpha reductase enzyme. Prostate-specific antigen blood tests and a digital rectal examination are useful in men over age 50 years to diagnose prostate cancer.

Erectile function testing may be appropriate in certain circumstances. If an investigation is required for clinical purposes where psychogenic aetiology is suspected (marked clinical indicators that are not recognized by the patient), consider use of a Rigiscan to measure nocturnal penile tumescence and rigidity (NPTR). A positive (normal) response can be enlightening for a man and will often allow the man to engage with psychosexual therapy (if recommended).

If an investigation is required for clinical purposes where neurological aetiology is suspected, refer for nerve conduction studies. The digital inflection rigidometer (DIR) test will assess distal rigidity in men complaining of 'soft tip' syndrome.

A variety of special investigations are available to provide more detailed understanding of the erectile process. These tests are of limited value in managing the majority of patients and should be reserved for selected patients such as those young men with ED secondary to blunt penile or perineal trauma.

Intracavernosal injection of a vasodilator (generally prostaglandin E1 or a combination of prostaglandin E1, papaverine and/or phentolamine) is used as a test to differentiate arterial inflow vasculogenic from venous leak vasculogenic ED. If after injection of the intracavernosal drug, a sustained erection is achieved then venous insufficiency is unlikely. If a full erection is not seen or if the erection lasts only a short time, the patient is allowed to stimulate himself in an attempt to improve the response. Patients with severe anxiety or needle phobia may not respond to this test. The integrity of the arterial perfusion pressure is not able to be assessed with the office intracavernosal injection test. A man with arterial insufficiency may still be able to achieve a functionally rigid erection with this test if the veno-occlusive mechanism is functioning satisfactorily. Arterial integrity is best assessed using a duplex Doppler examination or by directly recording cavernosal arterial perfusion pressure during dynamic pharmacocavernosometry.

Colour duplex Doppler ultrasound testing in conjunction with intracavernosal vasoactive agent injection may provide further information over injection alone in identifying vascular ED. This may be useful to a man with ED who is not yet aware that he may have an ongoing atherosclerotic process. If this test is positive, cardiovascular consultation may be indicated. After intracavernosal injection of a vasoactive agent, the penis can be scanned by a dorsal or ventral approach at the base, with the probe held transversely or in an oblique longitudinal position. The velocity of blood in the cavernosal artery during systolic and diastolic phases is recorded within 5 min of injection and repeated frequently. In general, peak systolic velocity values less than 30 cm/s are consistent with arterial pathology. A high resistance vascular bed, such as the engorged sinusoids of the erect penis, would only allow inflow during the high pressure systolic portion of the cardiac cycle. During diastole, the pressure would be insufficient to overcome the peripheral vascular resistance and the diastolic flow would be low (normally 3 cm/s and below).

Determination of the cavernosal artery systolic perfusion pressure and comparison of this value to the brachial artery systolic perfusion pressure is another method of determining arterial vascular integrity in selected patients. This procedure is best performed during dynamic pharmacocavernosometry. If the ED patient is young and has a history of blunt perineal/penile trauma with an intact veno-occlusive mechanism, reduced peak systolic velocity values (for his age) and reduced cavernosal artery systolic occlusion pressures, he becomes a candidate for selective internal pudendal arteriography, especially if he is considering undergoing the treatment option of microvascular arterial bypass surgery.

Investigations for men with problems of ejaculatory dysfunction

Men with rapid ejaculation should have a full clinical history documented (see Chapter 17) followed by a focused physical examination (especially indicated when the condition is acquired; and also in all cases before the prescription of any topical agents). A measure of TSH will exclude problems of thyroid function. Use of the (intravaginal ejaculation latency time) IELT may be helpful (stopwatch).

In men with delayed or inhibited ejaculation, following a clinical history (see Chapter 17), a physical examination is required of the testicles, epididymis, vasa, prostate and seminal vesicles. If the vasa are absent proceed to a renal scan to exclude cystic fibrosis. Confirm the presence or absence of the cremasteric (L1) and bulbocavernosus (S2-4) reflexes. Culture any expressed prostatic secretion in the urine after a DRE to exclude chronic prostatitis. Urine cytology may exclude any bladder carcinoma. Post-ejaculatory urinalysis is performed by centrifuging the post-ejaculatory urine specimen for 10 min any presence of sperm is suggestive of the diagnosis of retrograde ejaculation. In some cases, it may be prudent to proceed to ultrasonography of the testicles and epididymes or a CT scan with a full bladder. A trans-rectal ultrasound (TRUS) can identify any structural abnormalities such as ejaculatory duct stones, Mullerian duct cysts or dilatation of the seminal vesicles due to a stricture or other pathology.

Investigations for men with problems of dyspareunia

Following a detailed clinical history (see Chapter 19), the clinician should exclude any painful ejaculation and haemospermia that would require urological assessment. Exclusion of a sexually transmitted infection (STI) at a GU clinic may be indicated. Physical examination as outlined above should be conducted by a physician. Ultrasound of the scrotum may be indicated. A CT without contrast will identify any genitourinary system calculi.

Conclusion

In the majority of cases, a physical examination and some laboratory investigations are indicated as part of the assessment process across the spectrum of clinical problems presenting in the field of sexual medicine. These should be undertaken by a physician in conjunction with non-physician colleagues.

Further reading

Bachmann, G.A., Rosen, R., Pinn, V.W. *et al.* (2006) A state-of-the-art consensus on definitions, diagnosis and management. *Journal of Reproductive Medicine*, **51** (**6**), 447–56.

Clayton, A.H., Goldfischer, E., Goldstein, I. *et al.* (2013) Validity of the decreased sexual desire screener for diagnosing hypoactive sexual desire disorder. *Journal of Sex and Marital Therapy*, **39**(**2**), 132–43.

DeRogatis, L., Rosen, R.C., Goldstein, I., Werneburg, B., Kempthorne-Rawson, J., Sand, M. (2012) Characterization of hypoactive sexual desire disorder (HSDD) in men. *Journal of Sexual Medicine*, **9**, 812–20.

Gelbard, M., Hellstrom, W.J.G., McMahon, C.G. *et al.* (2013). Baseline characteristics from an ongoing phase 3 study of collagenase clostridium histolyticum in patients with Peyronie's disease. *Journal of Sexual Medicine*, **10**, 2822–31.

Goldstein, A., Burrows, L., Goldstein, I. (2010) Can oral contraceptives cause vestibulodynia? *Journal of Sexual Medicine*, **7**(**4 Pt 1**), 1585–7.

Goldstein, I. (2010) Recognizing and treating urogenital atrophy in postmenopausal women. *J Womens Health (Larchmt)*, **19**(**3**), 425–32.

Goldstein, I. (2007) A clinical paradigm for the combined management of androgen insufficiency and erectile dysfunction. *Endocrinology of Metabolism Clinics of North America*, **36**(**2**), 435–52.

Goldstein, I., Lurie, A.L., Lubisich, J.P. (2007) Bicycle riding, perineal trauma, and erectile dysfunction: data and solutions. *Current Urology Reports*, **8**(**6**), 491–7.

Goldstein, I., Alexander, J.L. (2005) Practical Aspects in the Management of Vaginal Atrophy and Sexual Dysfunction in Perimenopausal and Postmenopausal Women. *Journal of Sexual Medicine*, **s3**, 154–165.

Isidori, A.M., Buvat, J., Corona, G. *et al.* (2014) A Critical Analysis of the Role of Testosterone in Erectile Function: From Pathophysiology to Treatment-A Systematic Review. *Europena Urology*, **65**, 99–112.

Jackson, G., Nehra, A., Miner, M. *et al.* (2013) The assessment of vascular risk in men with erectile dysfunction: the role of the cardiologist and general physician. *International Journal of Clinical Practice*, **67**, 1163–72.

Kottmel, A., Goldstein, I Vulvoscopy. (2012) *Journal of Sexual Medicine*, **9**(**12**), 2990–3.

Miner, M., Nehra, A., Jackson, G. *et al.* (2014) All men with vasculogenic erectile dysfunction require a cardiovascular workup. *American Journal of Medicine*, **127**(**3**), 174–82.

Montorsi, F., Adaikan, G., Becher, E. *et al.* (2010) Summary of the recommendations on sexual dysfunctions in men. *Journal of Sexual Medicine*, **7**(**11**), 3572–88.

Mulhall, J., Althof, S.E., Brock, G.B., Goldstein, I., Junemann, K.P., Kirby, M. (2007) Erectile dysfunction: monitoring response to treatment in clinical practice–recommendations of an international study panel. *Journal of Sexual Medicine*, **4**(**2**), 448–64.

Nehra, A., Jackson, G., Miner, M. *et al.* (2012) The Princeton III Consensus Recommendations for the Management of Erectile Dysfunction and Cardiovascular Disease. *Mayo Clinic Proceedings*, **87**, 766–78.

Rosen, R.C., Maserejian, N.N., Connor, M.K., Krychman, M.L., Brown, C.S., Goldstein, I. (2012) Characteristics of premenopausal and postmenopausal women with acquired, generalized hypoactive sexual desire disorder: the Hypoactive Sexual Desire Disorder Registry for women. *Menopause*, **19**, 396–405.

Sommer, F., Goldstein, I., and Korda, J.B. (2010) Bicycle riding and erectile dysfunction: A review. *Journal of Sexual Medicine*, **7**(**7**), 2346–2358.

CHAPTER 11

Definition and Diagnosis of Sexual Problems

Johannes Bitzer

University Hospital Basel, Basel, Switzerland

OVERVIEW

- Sexual problems affect most men and women at least once during their lifetime and are thus part of the human condition
- Problems become clinical entities if the person cannot participate in a sexual relationship as he or she would wish, if this inability persist for a longer period of time and occurs in most attempts of being sexually active
- The main classification systems are ICD 10 by WHO and DSMIV/DSM-5 provided by the American Psychiatric Association
- ICD 10 is subdividing sexual problems into 4 groups distinguishing sexual dysfunctions, gender identity disorders, sexual preference disorders and Psychological and behavioural disorders associated with sexual development and orientation.
- DSM-5 differentiates between 3 groups of sexual problems namely sexual dysfunction, gender dysphoria and paraphilic disorders

What is a sexual problem?

A problem is an obstacle, which hinders the achievement of a particular goal, purpose or an objective.

A sexual problem is, according to the above definition, an obstacle to achieve the individual's desired sexual experience. There is a discrepancy between the sexual reality and the sexual ideal or in other words the subject's experience does not match the expectations. Taken this definition, it can be assumed that all human beings at least once during the lifetime have a sexual problem.

But when does a problem become a medical issue?

Example 1 John is 16 years old. He is deeply in love with Julie. She does not respond to his advances and therefore his strong desire for intimacy is frustrated and he is distressed and sad that he cannot express and live his sexual fantasies and dreams.

Is John exposed to an experience which is part of human life or is this a 'medical issue'?

Example 2 Frank is 63 years old. He has been married to Mary for 35 years. For about a year, Frank has noticed that when he wants to have intercourse with his wife, his penis is not getting as hard it did before, and that during intercourse the hardness is not maintained so that he may not have an orgasm. This distresses him and his wife and has lead to some avoidant behaviour towards sex in both partners.

Does Frank experience normal ageing or is this a 'medical issue'?

Example 3 Claire is 46 years old. For some time she has lost interest in any sexual activity. When her husband wants to have sex with her she tries to avoid intimacy. In the rare moments when she feels desire her body responds like before, and she can occasionally experience orgasm. She would like to feel more desire and enjoyment of sex, not only to please her husband but also to feel more younger and more 'like a woman'.

Is lack of motivation for sex a medical issue?

Example 4 Since puberty, Alice had felt that she was living in the wrong body. She hated her breasts developing and her hips getting broader. She trained very hard to get a 'six pack' abdomen. She did not feel like a girl and preferred to play soccer with boys. She does not exactly know whether she is more attracted to girls or to boys.

Is this just a developmental problem or a medical issue?

Example 5 In the metro, when close to a female passenger, Peter intermittently feels the urge to rub himself against the woman's body. This urge is so strong that he risks being accused in public.

Is this just bad behaviour or a medical issue?

From these examples, it can be seen that **sexual problems** may manifest themselves in different forms and at very different levels:

1. Sexual desire is frustrated and unfulfilled.
2. The body does not function sexually.
3. There is a loss of sexual motivation and interest.
4. The body has sex-specific characteristics (male/female), which are opposite to how the person feels about his or her sex (female/male).
5. The sexual behaviour of the person poses a problem to others or to the society in general.

The classification systems

There are two major classification systems for sexual disorders, namely the International Classification of Disease by the World

ABC of Sexual Health, Third Edition. Edited by Kevan Wylie.
© 2015 John Wiley & Sons, Ltd. Published 2015 by John Wiley & Sons, Ltd.

Table 11.1 Categories of sexual problems in the ICD-10

F52 Sexual dysfunction, not caused by organic disorder or disease
F52.0 Lack or loss of sexual desire
F52.1 Sexual aversion and lack of sexual enjoyment
10   Sexual aversion
11   Lack of sexual enjoyment
F52.2 Failure of genital response
F52.3 Orgasmic dysfunction
F52.4 Premature ejaculation
F52.5 Non-organic vaginismus
F52.6 Non-organic dyspareunia
F52.7 Excessive sexual drive
F52.8 Other
F52.9 Unspecified sexual dysfunction, not caused by organic disorder or disease

F64 Gender identity disorders
F64.0 Transsexualism
F64.1 Dual-role transvestism
F64.2 Gender identity disorder of childhood
F64.8 Other gender identity disorders
F64.9 Gender identity disorder, unspecified

F65 Disorders of sexual preference
F65.0 Fetishism
F65.1 Fetishistic transvestism
F65.2 Exhibitionism
F65.3 Voyeurism
F65.4 Paedophilia
F65.5 Sadomasochism
F65.6 Multiple disorders of sexual preference
F65.8 Other disorders of sexual preference
F65.9 Disorder of sexual preference, unspecified

F66 Psychological and behavioural disorders associated with sexual development and orientation
F66.0 Sexual maturation disorder
F66.1 Egodystonic sexual orientation
F66.2 Sexual relationship disorder
F66.8 Other psychosexual development disorders
F66.9 Psychosexual development disorder, unspecified

Source: WHO, 1993. Reproduced with permission from the World Health Organization.

Table 11.2 DSM-5 Classification

302.74	(F52.32)	Delayed ejaculation
	ICD-10	
302.72	(F52.21)	Erectile disorder
302.73	(F52.31)	Female orgasmic disorder
302.72	(F52.22)	Female sexual interest/arousal disorder
302.76	(F52.6)	Genito-pelvic pain Penetration disorder
302.71	(F52.0)	Male hypoactive sexual desire disorder
302.75	(F52.4)	Premature early ejaculation
302.79	(F52.8)	Other specified sexual dysfunction
302.70	(F52.9)	Unspecified sexual dysfunction
Gender dysphoria		
302.6	(F64.2)	Gender dysphoria in children
302.85	(F64.1)	Gender dysphoria in adolescents and adults
302.6	(F64.8)	Other specified gender dysphoria
302.6	(F64.9)	Unspecified gender dysphoria
Paraphilic disorder		
302.82	(F65.3)	Voyeuristic disorder
302.4	(F65.2)	Exhibitionistic disorder
302.89	(F65.81)	Frotteuristic disorder
302.83	(F65.51)	Sexual masochism disorder
302.84	(F65.52)	Sexual sadism disorder
302.2	(F65.4)	Pedophilic disorder
302.81	(F65.0)	Fetishistic disorder
302.3	(F65.1)	Transvestic disorder
302.89	(F65.89)	Other specified paraphilic disorders
302.9	(F65.9)	Unspecified paraphilic disorder

Health Organization and the Multiaxial Diagnostic and Statistical Manual by the American Psychiatric Association.

Categories of sexual problems in the ICD-10

International classification of diseases (ICD)-10 is subdividing sexual problems into four groups distinguishing sexual dysfunctions, gender identity disorders, sexual preference disorders and psychological and behavioural disorders associated with sexual development and orientation (see Table 11.1).

The approach to sexual dysfunctions is mainly oriented along the linear model of Masters and Johnson (excitement, plateau, orgasm) with the addition of the concept of desire disorders. Dysfunctions of desire, genital response (corresponding to excitement) and orgasm are shared categories for males and females with sub-definitions for each sex. Sex-specific definitions are given for premature ejaculation, non-organic vaginism and non-organic dyspareunia.

Excessive sexual drive is not defined and is described as a research category.

In gender identity disorders, transsexualism is distinct from dual-role transvestism and childhood gender identity disorder.

Disorders of sexual preference include the classical paraphilias. Notable diagnostic entities are fetishistic transvestism, pedophilia and sadomasochism.

The category of psychological and behavioural disorders associated with sexual development and orientation includes egodystonic sexual orientation as a diagnostic entity.

Categories of Sexual problems in DSM-5

Diagnostic and statistical manual of mental disorders DSM-5 differentiates between three groups of sexual problems, namely sexual dysfunction, gender dysphoria and paraphilic disorders (Table 11.2).

Sexual dysfunctions are mainly descriptive categories along clinical entities. For males, desire disorder, erectile dysfunction and premature ejaculation are distinctive diagnoses already described by Masters and Johnson. For females, desire and arousal problems have been put together to one diagnostic category, while female orgasmic disorder is a gender-specific diagnosis. The 'new' category of genito-pelvic pain and penetration disorder overcomes difficult differentiations between vaginism and dyspareunia.

With respect to gender dysphoria, the main differentiation is between adolescent and adult dysphoria. Paraphilias are again the classical ones and in addition to ICD-10 froitterism and transvestic disorders are mentioned among the paraphilias.

The diagnosis of sexual dysfunctions

For the general practitioner, sexual dysfunctions are the most frequently found sexual problems among their patients.

The diagnosis of the sexual dysfunctions in practice is performed in three steps.

Step 1: Definition and Descriptive Diagnosis

For health care professionals in Europe, the descriptive diagnosis can best be based on ICD-10 criteria. It is useful to combine this part of ICD with some additional criteria as defined in DSM-5 (see below).

The general characteristics in ICD-10 are:

G1. The subject is unable to participate in a sexual relationship as he or she should wish.

G2. The dysfunction occurs frequently, but may be absent on some occasions.

G3. The dysfunction has been present for at least 6 months.

G4. Not entirely attributable to any of the other mental and behavioural disorders in ICD-10, physical disorders (such as endocrine disorder) or drug treatment.

The additional criteria taken from the DSM-5 are:

Lifelong. The disturbance has been present since the individual became sexually active.

Acquired. The disturbance began after a period of relatively normal sexual function.

Generalized. Not limited to certain types of stimulation, situations or partners.

Situational. Only occurs with certain types of stimulation, situations or partners.

Mild, moderate or severe distress over the symptoms.

According to the patient's history and examination, one or several of the following descriptive diagnoses can be made.

Lack or loss of sexual desire

- Lack or loss of sexual desire, manifest by diminution of seeking out sexual cues, thinking about sex with associated feelings of desire or appetite or sexual fantasies.
- Lack of interest in initiating sexual activity either with partner or as solitary masturbation, at a frequency clearly lower than expected, taking into account age and context, or at a frequency very clearly reduced from previous much higher levels.

Sexual aversion

- The prospect of sexual interaction with a partner produces sufficient aversion, fear or anxiety that sexual activity is avoided, or, if it occurs, is associated with strong negative feelings and an inability to experience any pleasure.
- Not due to performance anxiety (reaction to previous failure of sexual response).

Lack of sexual enjoyment

- Genital response (orgasm and/or ejaculation) all occur during sexual stimulation, but are not accompanied by pleasurable sensations or feelings of pleasant excitement.
- Absence of manifest and persistent fear or anxiety during sexual activity.

Failure of genital response

For men:

- Erection sufficient for intercourse fails to occur when intercourse is attempted.
- The dysfunction appears as one of the following:
  - Full erection occurs during the early stages of lovemaking but disappears or declines when intercourse is attempted (before ejaculation if it occurs).
  - Erection does occur but only at times when intercourse is not being considered.
  - Partial erection, insufficient for intercourse, occurs, but not full erection.
  - No penile tumescence occurs at all.

For women:

- Failure of genital response, experienced as failure of vaginal lubrication, together with inadequate tumescence of the labia.
- The dysfunction appears as one of the following:
  - General: lubrication fails in all relevant circumstances.
  - Lubrication may occur initially but fails to persist for long enough to allow comfortable penile entry.
  - Situational: lubrication occurs only in some situations (e.g. with one partner but not another, or during masturbation, or when vaginal intercourse is not being contemplated).

Orgasmic dysfunction

Orgasmic dysfunction (either absence or marked delay) appearing as one of the following:

Orgasm has never been experienced in any situation.

Orgasmic dysfunction has developed after a period of relatively normal response:

- general: orgasmic dysfunction occurs in all situations and with any partner;
- situational.

For women: Orgasm does occur in certain situations (e.g. when masturbating or with certain partners).

For men, one of the following can be applied:

(i) only during sleep, never during the waking state;

(ii) never in the presence of the partner;

(iii) in the presence of the partner but not within her vagina.

Premature ejaculation

Inability to delay ejaculation sufficiently to enjoy love making, manifest as either

- Occurrence of ejaculation before or very soon after vaginal entry (if a time limit is required: before or within 15 s of vaginal entry), or
- Ejaculation in absence of sufficient erection to make vaginal entry possible.

Not due to prolonged abstinence of sexual activity.

Non-organic vaginismus

Spasm of the perivaginal muscles sufficient to prevent penile entry or make it uncomfortable.

The dysfunction appears as one of the following:

- Normal response has never been experienced.
- Vaginismus has developed after a period of relatively normal response:

	Biomedical		Psychological		Socio-cultural
	Chronic diseases and Drugs	Hormonal factors	Intra-individual	Inter-personal	
Predisposing Distant Indirect					
Precipitating Factors Trigger					
Maintaining Proximate Direct					

Figure 11.1 The biopsychosocial working hypothesis for sexual dysfunctions

◦ When vaginal entry is not attempted, a normal sexual response may occur.

◦ Any attempt at sexual contact leads to generalized fear, and attempts to avoid vaginal entry (e.g. spasm of the adductor muscles of the thighs).

Non-organic dyspareunia

For women:

◦ Pain during sexual intercourse, experienced at the entry of the vagina, throughout or only when deep thrusting of the penis occurs.

◦ Not attributable to vaginismus or failure of lubrication.

◦ Dyspareunia due to organic pathology should be classified according to the underlying disorder.

For men:

◦ Pain or discomfort during sexual response. Careful recording should be established of the timing of the pain and the exact localization.

◦ Absence of local physical factors. If found, the dysfunction should be classified elsewhere.

Step 2: The explanatory working hypothesis

After having established the descriptive diagnosis by combining ICD and some DSM-5 criteria, the practitioner will have to explore the contributing factors to the problem based on the biopsychosocial model.

This model tries to integrate biological, psychological and social factors along a timeline differentiating between predisposing, precipitating and maintaining factors to help the health care professional and the patient to understand the problem and the contributing factors (Figure 11.1).

Step 3: Comprehensive Diagnosis

Combining the description and the working hypothesis, the health care professional can establish a comprehensive diagnosis which will serve as a basis for developing a therapeutic plan.

Further reading

American Psychiatric Association (2013) *Diagnostic and Statistical Manuel of Mental Disorders*, 5th edn. American Psychiatric Press, Washington, DC.

Bitzer, J., Giraldi, A. & Pfaus, J. (2013) Sexual desire and hypoactive sexual desire disorder in women. Introduction and overview. Standard operating procedure (SOP Part 1). *Journal of Sexual Medicine*, **10**, 36–49.

Bitzer, J., Giraldi, A. & Pfaus, J. (2013) A standardized diagnostic interview for hypoactive sexual desire disorder in women: standard operating procedure (SOP Part 2). *Journal of Sexual Medicine*, **10**, 50–7.

Brotto, L.A., Bitzer, J., Laan, E., Leiblum, S. & Luria, M. (2010) Women's sexual desire and arousal disorders. *Journal of Sexual Medicine*, **7**, 586–614.

Kaplan, H.S. (1977) Hypoactive sexual desire disorder. *Journal of Sex and Marital Therapy*, **3**, 3–9.

Lief, H.I. (1977) Inhibited sexual desire. *Med Aspects Hum Sex*, **7**, 94–5.

Masters, W.H. & Johnson, V.E. (1966) *Human sexual response*. Bantam Books, New York.

Masters, W.H. & Johnson, V.E. (1970) *Human Sexual Inadequacy*. Little Brown, Boston, MA.

World Health Organization. The ICD-10 International Classification of mental and behavioral disorders. Geneva 1993

CHAPTER 12

Psychiatric Disorders and Sexuality (Including Trauma and Abuse)

Richard Balon

Wayne State University School of Medicine, MI, USA

> **OVERVIEW**
> - Sexual dysfunction associated with mental illness, substance abuse and sexual trauma/abuse is difficult to manage and should be referred to a specialist
> - Many psychiatric disorders and psychotropic medications are associated with sexual dysfunction
> - The clinical interview is the cornerstone in establishing the diagnosis and management plan
> - The management of sexual dysfunction associated with mental illness, substance abuse and sexual trauma/abuse may address the possible underlying cause (using mostly psychotherapy and sex therapy, or removal of the possible causative agent) or address the sexual dysfunction symptomatologically (using various medications and antidotes).

Introduction

Many psychiatric disorders are associated with sexual dysfunctions. Impairment of sexual functioning in a person with mental illness could be possibly part of her/his mental illness symptomatology (e.g. lack of sexual desire in depression), adverse reaction to medication used for treatment of her/his mental illness (e.g. delayed ejaculation or anorgasmia associated with serotonergic antidepressants), result of substance abuse (e.g. low sexual desire due to chronic cocaine abuse), or due to chronic physical illness (either independent of mental illness or as a result of adverse reaction to medications used for mental illness, for example metabolic syndrome or diabetes mellitus due to some antipsychotics) and/or its treatment. Impairment of sexual functioning could, of course, occur due to one of these causes or a combination of two or more.

The exact diagnosis of the underlying cause of sexual impairment is not always possible and thus treatment may either target the underlying cause, or be symptomatic, for example using treatments that work for a specific sexual dysfunction in general (e.g. using medication such as sildenafil (Viagra) for erectile dysfunction). The diagnosis is usually established during a careful clinical interview. The clinician has to ask very specific questions focused on particular parts of sexual functioning, for example on sexual desire,

arousal (erection), orgasm (ejaculation) and pain associated with sexual activity. It is imperative to obtain a baseline evaluation of the patient's sexual functioning during the first visit. This will be helpful later, in cases of sexual dysfunction possibly associated with any medication prescribed. There are no specific tests for sexual dysfunction(s). However, certain laboratory tests may help in some clinical situations. For instance, measuring the level of prolactin may help confirm suspected sexual dysfunction during the treatment with an antipsychotic drug.

Psychiatric disorders associated with sexual dysfunction(s)

Impairment or change in sexual functioning may occur during the course of almost any psychiatric disorder.

Mood disorders and sexual functioning

The most common complaint of depressed patients is decreased libido (up to 72% of patients in one study). It seems that the more severe the depression, the greater the loss of libido. Impairment of other aspects of sexual functioning, for example erectile dysfunction, impaired arousal in women, delayed ejaculation/orgasm and anorgasmia have also been reported in depressed individuals, although less frequently than decreased libido. Depressed individuals may also be anxious and anxiety is also associated with impairment of sexual functioning. It is important to note that while their sexual functioning may be impaired, good sexual functioning is important for them. The situation is also complicated by the fact that most medications used to treat depression have been associated with sexual dysfunction (see Table 12.1).

Changes of sexual functioning also occur frequently in bipolar patients – 30–65% of manic patients may display hypersexuality, while some may report decreased libido. Some patients suffering from bipolar or cyclothymic disorder (mild depression and hypomania) may also report episodes of promiscuity or extra relationship affairs.

Anxiety disorders and sexual functioning

As already noted, persons with high level of anxiety frequently have higher rates of impaired sexual functioning. Increased frequency

ABC of Sexual Health, Third Edition. Edited by Kevan Wylie.
© 2015 John Wiley & Sons, Ltd. Published 2015 by John Wiley & Sons, Ltd.

Table 12.1 Antidepressants reportedly associated with sexual dysfunctions in case reports and or studies

- Heterocyclics (amitriptyline, amoxapine, clomipramine, desipramine, doxepin, imipramine, nortriptyline, protriptyline, trimipramine, trazodone)
- Selective serotonin reuptake inhibitors (citalopram, escitalopram, fluoxetine, fluvoxamine, paroxetine, sertraline, vortioxetine[a])
- Monoamine oxidase inhibitors (isocarboxazid, moclobemide[a], phenelzine, selegiline[a], tranylcypromine)
- Other (agomelatine[a], bupropion[a], desvenlafaxine, duloxetine, levomilnacipran[a], milnacipran, mirtazapine[a], nefazodone[a], reboxetine[a], venlafaxine)

[a]Medications with claimed lower frequency of associated sexual dysfunction (most data probably on bupropion, mirtazapine and nefazodone).

of sexual problems has been reported in patient suffering from generalized anxiety disorder, panic disorder, obsessive–compulsive disorder, posttraumatic stress disorder and social phobia. Lower libido has been the most frequently reported dysfunction.

Schizophrenia and sexual dysfunction

Sexual dysfunction(s) in patients with schizophrenia occurs frequently. It may occur even before the onset of psychosis and any treatment. It also occurs in patients in remission. Impaired libido is usually the most frequently reported sexual problem. Some patients with chronic schizophrenia are known to masturbate excessively (we do not know the reason). The evaluation of sexual functioning in schizophrenia may be complicated by the patient's delusions, either of sexual or paranoid nature. As noted, some antipsychotic medications may be associated with impaired sexual functioning probably due to the increased levels of prolactin secondary to the use of these medications.

Other psychiatric disorders and sexual functioning

Examples of other psychiatric disorders associated with impaired sexual functioning include eating disorders (e.g. anorexia – low sexual desire, fear of intimacy, inhibited sexual behaviour; decreased frequency of masturbation and intercourse), personality disorders (e.g. borderline personality disorder) and more controversially obstructive sleep apnoea (e.g. erectile dysfunction).

Substance abuse and sexual functioning

Changes of sexual functioning may occur during substance use and abuse of various drugs of abuse. Some drugs may increase sexual response in the early stages of use, chronic use usually leads to impairment of all aspects of sexual functioning, from decreased libido to impaired orgasm. For instance, alcohol is usually considered to be a social 'lubricant', but intoxication interferes with erection, vaginal lubrication and orgasm. Chronic alcohol use may lead to chronic changes in sexual functioning due to testicular atrophy in men and reduction of oestradiol in women, which can be associated with impaired lubrication and dyspareunia. Other drugs reported to be associated with sexual dysfunction(s) are opioids (chronic use – all aspects of sexual

functioning may be impaired), stimulants/cocaine (acute use is associated with sexual enhancement, while chronic use may lead to erectile dysfunction and delayed orgasm). Cannabis may be associated with increased sexual satisfaction and pleasure during acute use, the effects of its chronic use have not been properly studied. Ecstasy (3,4-methylenedioxy-methamphetamine (MDMA)) may increase desire and satisfaction, but inhibits orgasm. One should not forget that tobacco smoking has a negative impact on sexual functioning, as nicotine is a potent vasoconstrictor (thus, frequent erectile dysfunction in male smokers).

Trauma and sexual functioning

Sexual trauma, either in childhood or in adulthood, has frequently a profound impact on adult sexual functioning. There are several dimensions of sexual trauma that may influence a person's sexual functioning, such as the type of sexual trauma and related variables (e.g. violent vs. non-violent trauma; being abused by a close person), the way sexual trauma was dealt with at the time it happened (disclosed? secret? shame?), and the way the abused person views it at the present. The distrust resulting from trauma may lead to impairment of emotional and sexual intimacy and then result in lack of sexual desire and avoidance. Sexual trauma and/or abuse may result in other sexual dysfunctions, such as lack of arousal, anorgasmia and pain during sexual activity.

Evaluation

One has to obtain a detailed evaluation of both sexual functioning and mental illness/substance abuse/sexual trauma before addressing the sexual dysfunction. Unfortunately, we do not have many specific tests for evaluating sexual dysfunctions, with the exception of a few tests for evaluating erectile functioning (e.g. nocturnal phaloplethysmography or NPT) or levels of some hormones (prolactin, testosterone). Thus, a detailed, thorough clinical interview is usually the cornerstone of the evaluation.

The part of the interview focusing on sexual functioning should establish whether there really is sexual dysfunction present, which one it is (low sexual desire? impaired arousal? both?) and whether there is a temporal relationship between the mental disorder/substance abuse/sexual trauma and impaired sexual functioning. It may not be always easy to establish the temporal relationship. However, it is important to realize that the sexual dysfunction may be independent of the mental illness/substance abuse or trauma, or that some symptomatology of mental illness (e.g. depressed mood) may occur in response to preexisting sexual dysfunction.

The baseline evaluation of sexual functioning is especially important within the framework of sexual dysfunction associated with various medications (e.g. antidepressants, antipsychotics, drugs used to treat hypertension, drugs used to treat cancer).

It is important that both the patient and the clinician feel comfortable talking about sex. This may not always be easy in patients with some mental illnesses. A depressed or traumatized patient may not be willing to discuss sex in details or at all, while a hypomanic patient may try to share every detail of her/his sexual functioning.

Table 12.2 Laboratory test useful for evaluating sexual dysfunction (always consider clinical situation)

Recommended	Optional
Testosterone (free and total)	Fasting glucose
Thyroid-stimulating hormone (TSH)	Glycosylated haemoglobin A_{1C}
Prolactin	Lipid profile
Sex-hormone-binding globulin	Complete blood count
Oestradiol	Follicle-stimulating hormone, luteinizing Hormone, dehydroepiandrosterone

The atmosphere of the interview should be non-intrusive, comfortable, and the patient should feel that all information shared will remain confidential. The questioning should be semi-structured, with progressing to more specific questions about various aspects/parts of sexual functioning (libido, arousal, orgasm). One should always keep in mind the biopsychosocial model, asking about possible biological, psychological and social, or interpersonal aspects of sexual functioning. The clinician should not assume that because the patient suffers from mental illness, he/she is not interested in sex. For instance, it is known that many depressed patients desire 'normal' sexual functioning although their libido is low.

The evaluation should include a review of systems and possibly physical examination and laboratory testing, if indicated (Table 12.2). If possible, an interview with the patient's sexual partner should also be conducted.

Managing sexual dysfunction associated with mental illness, substance abuse or sexual trauma/abuse

Management of sexual dysfunction in the context of coexisting mental illness, substance abuse or sexual trauma is complex and difficult. The primary goal – treatment or removal of the underlying condition – is not always possible and may be counterproductive for the treatment of the underlying conditions.

Management may start with removal of the possible causative agent in cases of sexual dysfunction associated with treatment of mental illness or with substances of abuse. As stopping medication is not always possible, various strategies developed especially in the area of sexual dysfunction associated with antidepressants may be implemented (Table 12.3). The clinician should always attempt to address modifiable risks, such as obesity, smoking and should try to implement a diet (e.g. Mediterranean) and exercise.

Suggesting a modified approach to sexual activity – for example deferring intercourse and orgasm while focusing on sensual, non-genital pleasure and intimacy, or suggesting non-coital options for achieving orgasm (including helping the partner achieve orgasm even if the patient is not able, and using sexual aids (vibrators, vacuum pumps – there is a small vacuum pump available for women, too – EROS clitoral therapy device)) – may be helpful. Involving the partner in the management may be quite helpful and may involve discussing different approaches to sex,

Table 12.3 Strategies for medication-associated sexual dysfunction

- Primarily selecting an agent with a lower frequency of sexual dysfunction (e.g. bupropion, mirtazapine among antidepressants, second-generation antipsychotics with the exception of risperidone)
- Waiting for spontaneous remission of sexual dysfunction (not frequent, difficult for the patient to implement at times)
- Reducing the dose (not always possible, symptomatology of mental illness may reappear)
- Scheduling medication in relation to sexual activity (e.g. taking the entire daily dose after evening sex, not always helpful)
- Drug holidays (i.e. stopping medication for 2–3 days, sexual activity at the end of this interval and then resuming medication; questionable approach not usually recommended)
- Switching to medications with lower frequency of sexual dysfunction (e.g. bupropion and mirtazapine among antidepressants, second-generation antipsychotics with the exception of risperidone)
- Using various 'antidotes' including the PDE-5i, vacuum erectile devices or prosthesis

implementing alternative coital positions, avoiding sexual activity during conflicts, when fatigued and so on.

Psychotherapy and sex therapy are the mainstay and should be implemented whenever possible. Cognitive-behavioural therapy should be used for anxiety, depression and other mental illnesses whenever possible. Some patients, especially those with a history of sexual trauma/abuse may require intensive, long-term individual therapy.

At times, pharmacotherapy for sexual dysfunction associated with mental illness or substances may be used. Phosphodiesterase-5 inhibitors (PDE-5is) such as avanafil, sildenafil, tadalafil and vardenafil may be helpful in erectile dysfunction associated with mental illness (e.g. depression) or medications (antidepressants, antipsychotics). Occasionally, PDE-5i were found useful even in women with impaired sexual function due to antidepressants. Adding the antidepressant bupropion may occasionally help in cases of low sexual desire (especially in depressed patients). Using hormones, such as testosterone in men, should be limited to cases of clearly established hypogonadism. Sexual dysfunction due to various psychotropic medications may be alleviated by numerous antidotes (Table 12.4).

Various treatment modalities could certainly be combined, for example sex therapy with PDE5i.

Table 12.4 Antidotes used to manage sexual dysfunction associated with medications

Amantadine	Methylphenidate
Bethanechol	Mirtazapine
Bupropion	Mianserin
Buspirone	Nefazodone
Cyproheptadine	Neostigmine
Dextroampetamine	Pramipexol
Ephedrine	Ropinirole
Gingko biloba extract	Sildenafil and other PDE5i
Granisetron	Trazodone
Loratadine	Yohimbine

These antidotes are used for various dysfunctions and with various frequencies. The evidence is mostly based on case reports or case series, although a few controlled studies exist.

Further reading

Balon, R. (2006) SSRI-associated sexual dysfunction. *American Journal of Psychiatry*, **163**, 1504–1509.

Casper, R.C., Redmond, D.E., Katz, M.M., Schaffer, C.B., Davis, Z.J.M. & Koslow, S.H. (1985) Somatic symptoms in primary affective disorder. Presence and relationship to the classification of depression. *Archives of General Psychiatry*, **42**, 1098–1104.

Marques, T.R., Smith, S., Bonaccorso, S. *et al.* (2012) Sexual dysfunction in people with prodromal or first episode psychosis. *British Journal of Psychiatry*, **210**, 131–136.

McCarthy, B. & Farr, E. (2011) The impact of sexual trauma on sexual desire and function. *Advances in Psychosomatic Medicine*, **31**, 105–120.

Pacheco Palha, A. & Esteves, E. (2008) Drugs of abuse and sexual functioning. *Advances in Psychosomatic Medicine*, **29**, 131–149.

Seeman, M.V. (2013) Loss of libido in woman with schizophrenia. *American Journal of Psychiatry*, **170**, 471–475.

Stevenson, R. & Elliott, S. (2009) Sexual disorders with comorbid psychiatric or physical illness. In: Balon, R. & Segraves, R.T. (eds), *Clinical Manual of Sexual Disorders*. American Psychiatric Publishing, Inc., Arlington, VA, pp. 59–94.

Zemishlany, Z. & Weizman, A. (2008) The impact of mental illness on sexual function. *Advances in Psychosomatic Medicine*, **29**, 89–106.

CHAPTER 13

Medication and Sexual Dysfunction

John Dean

Clinical Director, Gender & Sexual Medicine, Devon Partnership NHS Trust, Exeter, UK

> **OVERVIEW**
> - The use of prescribed and recreational drugs should always be considered in the assessment of sexual dysfunction, although it is more typically the consequence of multiple contributory factors.
> - Drug effects are commonly cited as a cause of sexual dysfunction, but the evidence for this is limited and often anecdotal.
> - Underlying conditions for which drugs are prescribed may also cause or contribute to sexual dysfunction.
> - Commonly-used psychotropic drugs are amongst the most likely to be associated sexual dysfunction.
> - Cardiovascular disease is a more likely cause of sexual dysfunction than drugs used in its treatment.
> - Opiates, as well as several endocrine drugs, may cause testosterone deficiency and sexual dysfunction.

Introduction

Sexual dysfunction is typically the consequence of multiple contributory factors, rather than of one single factor. The use of prescribed medication and recreational drugs should always be considered in a comprehensive biopsychosocial assessment of sexual dysfunction in both men and women. Drug effects are commonly cited as a cause of sexual dysfunction, but the evidence for this is limited and often anecdotal. Underlying conditions for which drug treatments are prescribed may also cause or contribute to sexual dysfunction.

As a general rule, if there is a temporal relationship between the introduction of a new drug therapy, and the onset of a change in sexual response, or sexual dysfunction or dysfunctions, then it is more likely that the newly introduced drug is a causal or contributory factor; where a drug has been introduced more than a month before the onset of sexual symptoms, this is less likely. Prescribers should enquire about their patient's sexual function before they prescribe a drug known to be associated with sexual dysfunction; this information may lead them to prescribe a drug less likely to affect

Table 13.1 Strategies for the management of drug-induced sexual dysfunction

Strategy	Advantages	Disadvantages
Wait for accommodation	Simple	Low success rate
Reduce drug dose	Simple	Relapse of treated condition
Drug holiday	Avoids polypharmacy	Relapse of treated condition; non-compliance
Drug substitution	Avoids polypharmacy	Fear of relapse of treated condition
Specific antidotes	Good success with for some interventions (e.g. PDE5i for ED)	Polypharmacy; increased likelihood of side-effects; increased cost

sexual function in patients with pre-existing dysfunction, as well as helping them to more readily identify drug-induced dysfunction.

Strategies for the management of drug-induced sexual dysfunction are described in Table 13.1. These are mostly based on expert opinion and few have been evaluated in randomized, controlled trials; each has its advantages and disadvantages.

Whilst the prevention and amelioration of sexual dysfunction is important, this must be balanced against the effective treatment of the underlying condition for which the offending medication has been prescribed.

Psychotropic drugs

The relationship between psychiatric illness, its treatment and sexual dysfunction is complex and probably bidirectional. A patient's experience of altered sexual response may be the result of pre-existing sexual dysfunction, a symptom of depression and anxiety, an undesirable side-effect of the psychotropic medication, or a consequence of other medical problems, substance misuse, or psychosocial and relationship stress.

Antipsychotic medication

Sexual problems are common amongst people with psychosis as well as amongst those taking antipsychotic drugs; compliance may

---

ABC of Sexual Health, Third Edition. Edited by Kevan Wylie.
© 2015 John Wiley & Sons, Ltd. Published 2015 by John Wiley & Sons, Ltd.

be compromised by sexual problems that affected persons associate with their use of antipsychotic medication, whether medication is the true cause or not. Sex and relationship problems may result from emotional dysregulation associated with psychosis.

All types of sexual dysfunctions (decreased libido, impaired arousal/erection, retrograde ejaculation, delayed ejaculation, priapism and others) have been reported to be associated with antipsychotic medications. Antipsychotics that increase prolactin are associated with more reports of sexual problems than those which do not. Dose-related hyperprolactinaemia is seen with first-generation antipsychotic medications, and amisulpride and risperidone. It has been calculated that around 40% of treatment-emergent sexual side-effects in schizophrenia are attributable to the prolactin-raising properties of antipsychotic medication. Of these attributable fraction, one- to two-thirds are attributable to hyperprolactinaemia. Despite increased prolactin, improved emotional regulation, as a consequence of effective treatment with antipsychotic drugs, may improve sexual function.

Prolactin increases within hours of initiation of treatment with a relevant drug and continues whilst treatment is maintained. In long-term treatment, there may be a gradual decrease in prolactin but it remains elevated in most patients. If oral treatment is withdrawn, prolactin returns to normal range within 2–3 weeks, depending on the half-life of the drug and its metabolites; it may remain elevated for 6 months after discontinuation of intramuscular depot preparations.

No change, or a slight decrease, in prolactin is usually seen with olanzapine, quetiapine, aripiprazole and clozapine. The atypical antipsychotics, with the exception of amisulpride and risperidone, are associated with fewer reports of sexual side-effects. Whilst clozapine has little effect on prolactin, reports of sexual dysfunction associated with its use are also common.

Both the initiation and withdrawal of antipsychotics have been associated with persistent genital arousal disorder (PGAD), a rare condition characterized by spontaneous, unrelenting and distressing genital arousal in women not linked to sexual desire. It may be analogous to priapism (rigid erection, persisting for 4 or more hours, in the absence of sexual stimulation) in men, which has also been associated with the use of antipsychotics. PGAD requires specialist assessment and treatment may be difficult. Priapism is a urological emergency, requiring immediate hospital referral and treatment.

Waiting for accommodation is rarely effective and not recommended for a patient who is bothered by sexual problems related to antipsychotic drugs. The use of olanzapine, quetiapine, aripiprazole and clozapine as first-line treatments, or their substitution for antipsychotics suspected of causing sexual dysfunction, should reduce the incidence of drug-related sexual dysfunction. Drug holidays increase the risk of a relapse of psychotic illness and are usually not appropriate.

In men with suspected antipsychotic-related erectile dysfunction (ED), consider prescribing a supply of at least eight sildenafil citrate 100 mg tablets, taken 'on demand' according to the manufacturer's instructions, in addition to their existing antipsychotic regimen, as a specific antidote. In men and women with low desire, other sexual dysfunction and/or hyperprolactinaemia, consider adding aripiprazole 15–30 mg/day to their existing antipsychotic

regimen. Several small studies have shown statistically significant improvements in sexual functioning or hyperprolactinaemia when aripiprazole was added to an existing antipsychotic regimen. Whilst aripiprazole is approved for the treatment of psychosis, it is not approved for the treatment of drug-related sexual dysfunction. There is inadequate evidence to support the use of other proposed antidotes, such as cyproheptadine and selegeline.

Cabergoline and bromocriptine should be considered for the treatment of severe hyperprolactinaemia (>735 min/l). This should first be discussed with an endocrinologist and the lowest effective dose prescribed; more intensive monitoring of the patient's mental health is mandatory, as this intervention may affect the efficacy of the causal antipsychotic drug. Severe hyperprolactinaemia, in the absence of sexual dysfunction, should also be treated, as it may lead to hypogonadism and other unwanted metabolic consequences. Hypogonadism is an important health problem, increasing risk from cardiovascular disease, depression, diabetes, obesity and osteoporosis and requires active management.

Antidepressants

In some studies, up to 90% of patients suffering from depression complained of reduced sexual desire; depression is also associated with other changes in sexual response, such as ED, decreased vaginal lubrication, and, particularly, delayed orgasm and anorgasmia. In a cross-sectional study of 6297 people with major depressive disorder on antidepressant monotherapy, 37% were identified as having sexual dysfunction by a validated questionnaire instrument. The selective serotonin re-uptake inhibitors (SSRIs), citalopram, fluoxetine, paroxetine and sertraline, as well as the Serotonin-noradrenaline reuptake inhibitor (SNRI), venlafaxine, did not differ from each other in prevalence of sexual dysfunction, suggesting a class effect of serotonin reuptake inhibitory medications.

Both the initiation and withdrawal of SSRIs have been associated with persistent PGAD in women. Tricyclic and monamine oxidase inhibitor antidepressants have been reported as causing sexual dysfunctions, including decreased libido, ED, and delayed and painful ejaculation. Clomipramine is particularly associated with delayed orgasm and anorgasmia. Trazodone is a rare cause of priapism.

Waiting for accommodation is not usually effective in resolving SSRI/SNRI-related sexual dysfunction. Reducing the dose of antidepressant to the minimum effective dose has been examined in one open-label study and was found useful only in medications with a shorter half-life, such as paroxetine and sertraline, and not in SSRIs with long half-life, such as fluoxetine. Expert opinion supports substitution of mirtazapine, reboxetine or agomelatine, which seem to have less impact on sexual function. Sildenafil may be used as a specific antidote for men affected by ED. Buspirone and bupropion have been studied as possible specific antidotes for SSRI/SNRI-related sexual dysfunction, but results have been conflicting; neither is approved for this indication.

Anxiolytics

Use of benzodiazepines is associated with reports of sexual dysfunction in women, possibly related to their sedating effect, but only rarely in men, possibly because of a reduction in performance anxiety. Buspirone is thought to have less effect on sexual response.

Opiates

Chronic opiate use may disrupt the hypothalmic–pituitary–gonadal axis and is associated with hypogonadism, which may result in sexual dysfunction. Behavioural and relationship disturbances, related to chronic opiate use, may also affect sexual and relationship satisfaction. Tramadol, a widely prescribed synthetic opiate, also has marked serotonergic activity and may additionally cause delayed orgasm or anorgasmia.

Cardiovascular drugs

Cardiovascular drugs may provoke changes in sexual response by a variety of mechanisms, including haemodynamic, neurotransmitter, hormonal and psychological effects and through more general side-effects, such as fatigue and dry mouth. Cardiovascular disease may, in itself, cause sexual dysfunction through a variety of mechanisms. Patients affected by heart failure and coronary artery disease may experience fatigue and depression; they (and their partners) may fear that the exertion associated with sex may be dangerous, and that drug treatments for sexual dysfunction might add to their risk.

The prevalence of ED in untreated hypertension has been reported as 17%, and 25% in treated hypertension. In a study of treated hypertensive women over 60, 50% experienced sexual dysfunction: 25% reported delayed or absent orgasm; 23% reported lubrication problems; 15% reported reduced libido. The risk of having sexual dysfunction amongst people with hypertension is increased by the use of multiple antihypertensive agents.

The evidence that thiazide diuretics cause sexual dysfunction is conflicting, with studies reporting an incidence ranging from 0% to 31%; ED is the most commonly reported problem.

Angiotensin-converting enzyme inhibitor (ACE-inhibitor) and calcium channel blockers seem to have little effect on sexual function and are not commonly associated with ED.

Alpha-blockers also seem to have little effect on erection but, as a class, they are associated with retrograde ejaculation, which may be distressing for some men. They are associated with rare reports of priapism.

Several studies suggest that angiotensin receptor blockers (ARBs, sartans) have a positive effect on erectile function in hypertensive men. There is a reasonable argument for them to be used as first-line therapy for hypertension in men with pre-existing ED, and there is also some evidence that they have less effect on sexual response in women.

The non-selective beta-blockers propranolol is associated with sexual dysfunctions, including ED and reduced desire. This is much less common in more selective beta-blockers, such as atenolol.

Spironolactone is an androgen receptor antagonist and commonly causes sexual effects associated with reduced androgen action, such as low desire and ED.

Drugs for lower urinary tract symptoms

Men with lower urinary tract symptoms (LUTSs), untreated by drugs, are more likely to report sexual dysfunctions, particularly ED, anejaculation and retrograde and premature ejaculation than the general population. Drugs used for the treatment of LUTS may also cause sexual dysfunctions.

Alpha-blockers

Alpha-blockers, used for the treatment of LUTS and hypertension, are associated with 'dry' orgasm in men (retrograde or anejaculation), with a reported incidence of up to 30%. Ejaculatory dysfunction may be more common with the 1-alpha selective drug tamsulosin than with the non-selective drugs alfuzosin, terazosin and doxazosin. Ejaculatory dysfunction rapidly resolves when the alpha-blocker is withdrawn.

5-alpha reductase inhibitors

The 5-alpha reductase inhibitors finasteride and dutasteride are treatments for benign prostatic hyperplasia; finasteride is also used for the treatment of androgenic alopecia. They block the conversion of testosterone to dihydrotestosterone, a more potent androgen. Both drugs are associated with ED, reduced desire, ejaculatory dysfunction and reduced semen quality, with an incidence of up to 40%. For most men, these side-effects resolve a few weeks after the drug is withdrawn but around 2% of users experience persistent sexual dysfunction that may continue for months or even years after discontinuation. The mechanism for this is unclear but it may be related to changes in neurosteroid metabolism within the brain.

Endocrine drugs

Anti-androgens

Anti-androgens, typically used in the treatment of prostate cancer are associated with ED and reduced sexual desire; the likely mechanism is a reduction in androgen action, both in the central nervous system (CNS) and peripherally. Gonadotrophin-releasing hormone agonists seem to have a greater effect on sexual function than the non-steroidal anti-androgen, bicalutamide. The sexual side-effects of these drugs may persist for many months after their withdrawal and some effects may be permanent. PDE5i drugs may be tried as a specific antidote for ED but men using anti-androgens are less responsive.

Anti-oestrogens

The anti-oestrogen tamoxifen and aromatase inhibitor anastrozole are both associated with vaginal dryness and dyspareunia, as a consequence of reduced oestrogen effect on the vaginal mucosa. Some women benefit from the use of longer-acting water- and silicone-based lubricants, although their use does not always restore pleasurable sensation. Affected women may be deeply distressed by resulting impairment of sexual function, which is difficult to resolve; some may seek referral to a specialist centre for consideration of topical oestrogen therapy, despite the risk of cancer recurrence.

Hormonal contraception

The sexual side-effects of hormonal contraceptives are not well-studied. There appear to be mixed effects on libido, with a minority of women experiencing an increase or a decrease, and the majority being unaffected. There is evidence that ethinyl oestradiol provokes a long-lasting or permanent increase in sex hormone binding globulin production, reducing free testosterone; the clinical relevance of this is unclear. It is suggested that this may cause long-lasting reduced sexual desire in women.

Lipid-lowering drugs

Evidence of an effect of lipid-lowering statin and fibrate drugs on erectile function is mixed. These drugs tend to improve endothelial function and there is some evidence of a synergistic effect on erection quality with PDE5i drugs. However, they are also associated with lower testosterone levels. On the balance of current evidence, lipid-lowering drugs do not seem to have a significant negative impact on sexual function.

Further reading

Clayton, A.H. & Balon, R. (2009) The Impact of mental illness and psychotropic medications on sexual functioning: The evidence and management. *The Journal of Sexual Medicine*, **6**, 1200–1211.

Hackett, G. (2011) Cardiovascular drugs and sexual dysfunction. *Primary Care Cardiovascular Journal*, **4**(**3**), 124–126.

Maggi, M., Buvat, J., Corona, G., Guay, A. & Torres, L.O. (2013) Hormonal causes of male sexual dysfunctions and their management (hyperprolactinemia, thyroid disorders, GH disorders, and DHEA). *The Journal of Sexual Medicine*, **10**(**3**), 661–77.

Montorsi, F., Basson, R., Adaikan, G., *et al.* (2010) *Sexual Medicine, Sexual Dysfunctions in Men and Women*. Health Publications Ltd.

CHAPTER 14

Problems of Sexual Desire in Men

Yacov Reisman[1] and Francesca Tripodi[2]

[1]Men's Health Clinics – Amstelland Hospital, Amstelveen and Bovenij Hospital, Amsterdam, The Netherlands
[2]Institute of Clinical Sexology, Rome, Italy

OVERVIEW

- Hypoactive sexual desire disorder (HSDD) in men is recognized as the most difficult sexual disorder to define, evaluate and treat
- The detection of HSDD in men is not difficult if the clinician asks directly about desire, interest or wish for sexual activity
- The history is crucial step in correct diagnosis and exploring the causes
- Bio-psycho-social causes often mutually interact in determining HSDD
- Treatment of HSDD should be etiologically oriented
- Treatment aims to encourage the recreational and hedonistic aspect of sexuality and on improving communication between partners.

Introduction

Although there are large number of studies on hypoactive sexual desire disorder (HSDD) in women, research on HSDD in men is scarce. Furthermore, many men are treated for different sexual diagnoses while they are suffering from HSDD. The lack of education on sexual issues, the myth that men are always motivated for sexual activities and lack of effective clinical tools to asses HSDD contribute to these misdiagnoses.

Sexual desire is the result of a positive interplay among internal cognitive processes (thoughts, fantasy and imagination), neurophysiological mechanisms (central arousability) and affective components (mood and emotional states), the biological basis of which is almost unknown in humans.

Although no broad consensus exists regarding an accepted definition for sexual desire, in an attempt to capture its complex nature, Levine define desire as 'the motivation or inclination to be *sexual*' and suggests that this construct be considered in terms of the following components which link several different theoretical perspectives together:

- *Drive*: The biological component. This includes anatomy and neuroendocrine physiology.

- *Motivation*: The psychological component. This includes the influences of personal mental states (mood), interpersonal states (e.g. mutual affection, disagreement) and social context (e.g. relationship status).
- *Wish*: The cultural component. This considers cultural ideals, values and rules about sexual expressions which are external to the individual.

Definitions of low sexual desire in men

Low sexual desire in men is one of the most difficult sexual disorders to define, evaluate and treat. The main problem is the lack of a definition that is widely accepted. According to the classification of the *Diagnostic and statistical manual of mental disorders* (DSM-5), male HSDD is considered a sexual dysfunction and is characterized as a persistent or recurrent lack (or absence) of sexual fantasies and desire for sexual activity, as judged by a clinician taking into account factors that affect sexual functioning (e.g. age, general and socio-cultural contexts of the individual's life). Symptoms have persisted for a minimum of 6 months. The disturbance must cause marked distress or severe interpersonal difficulties; cannot be better accounted for by another major mental disorder (except another sexual dysfunction); and is not due solely to the effects of a substance or general medical condition.

HSDD, as defined by DSM, has garnered much criticism. The main problem is that the concept of sexual desire is poorly defined in this diagnosis as well as in the current literature.

Disorders such as depression or erectile dysfunction frequently coexist with low sexual desire. In addition, the DSM definition is based on the traditional model of human sexual response derived from the work of Helen Singer Kaplan, with her *linear* model which also ignores the differences between male and female sexuality. It is now recognized that sexual desire can be responsive, occurring after arousal or physical stimulation, rather than a spontaneous event before arousal. Hence, recent approaches conceptualize sexual desire as a predisposition to respond subjectively to sexual stimuli with feelings of sexual arousal, suggesting that sexual desire is the cognitive valence of sexual arousal. Accordingly, recent studies found that sexual desire and sexual arousal are overlapping constructs as both depend on the ability of an individual to process sexual information during sexual activity.

ABC of Sexual Health, Third Edition. Edited by Kevan Wylie.
© 2015 John Wiley & Sons, Ltd. Published 2015 by John Wiley & Sons, Ltd.

Relationship dimensions, psychological adaptation, cognitive factors and biological determinants have all been related to sexual desire.

Very recently, in 2013, a new classification scheme has been suggested by Rubio-Aurioles *et al.*: *Low Sexual Desire/Interest* (LSD/I) as an umbrella term for which HSDD is only a subtype, to refer to the clinical condition where the man complains about a modification in his usual level of sexual interest or desire and therefore is presented as a condition that can be best characterized as a syndrome rather than a disorder. The definition for LSD/I is:

'diminished or absent feelings of sexual interest or desire, absent sexual thoughts or fantasies and lack of a responsive desire. Motivations (defined as reasons/incentives) for attempting to become sexually aroused are scarce or absent'

In addition, the presence of personal or interpersonal distress has been suggested as a requisite to justify clinical intervention in sexual dysfunction. As the coexistence of LSD/I with other sexual dysfunctions is rather common, the International Society for Sexual Medicine propose to use the term LSD/I as a general term for the symptom/syndrome that might be caused by medical conditions such as depression or endocrine abnormalities, relationship factors, medications or drugs abuse and to reserve the DSM V-TR HSDD for the cases where other etiological factors have been appropriately excluded.

Epidemiology

HSDD has been historically either not identified or erroneously diagnosed and presented as another sexual dysfunction such as erectile dysfunction. The most important population-based studies report that the prevalence of reduced sexual interest ranges from 3% to more than 50%. Interestingly, the populations' level of sexual interest appears quite stable from the late teens and up to about 60, thereafter it decreases markedly.

In a multicentre survey study involving 374 men (mean age 48.8 years), recruited for a pharmaceutical study, 30% met the DSM criteria for HSDD as a primary diagnosis. A survey conducted in the United States in 2004 involving 1455 men aged 57–85 years showed 28% of men reported lack of desire, with 65% of them feeling bothered about it. According to expert opinion, it seems to be that the acquired and situational form of HSDD is the most common subtype for men.

Aetiology

In general, men are diagnosed with one of three subtypes of HSDD/LSD:

- *Lifelong/generalized*: The man has little or no desire for sexual stimulation (with a partner or alone) and never had.
- *Acquired/generalized*: The man previously had sexual interest with his current partner, but lacks interest in sexual activity, partnered or solitary.
- *Acquired/situational*: The man was previously sexually interested with his current partner but now lacks sexual interest in him/her but has desire for sexual stimulation (i.e. alone or with someone other than his current partner).

Table 14.1 Common factors associated with HSDD in Men

Hormonal
Androgen deficiency
Hyperprolactinemia
Psychological
Anger and anxiety
Depression
Relationship conflicts
Post-traumatic stress syndrome
Eating disorders
Chronic disease
Cardiovascular accidents
Epilepsy
Renal failure
Coronary disease and heart failure
Ageing
HIV
Medications (see Table 14.2) and lifestyle
Antidepressant therapy
Bodybuilding and eating disorders

Source: Adapted from Corona *et al.* 2013 Reproduced with permission from Medix.

Biological, intra-psychic and marital factors (biopsychosocial causes) often mutually interact in determining HSDD/LSD. In many cases, the cause of HSDD is simply unknown. Therefore, research exploring sexual desire suggests that it may be related to any number of sexually specific and nonspecific factors (see Table 14.1).

Determinants of **lifelong/generalized HSDD** is more frequently uncertain.

In the case of **acquired/generalized low sexual desire**, possible causes include low levels of testosterone (T) or high levels of prolactin (PRL), various medical/health problems, and psychiatric problems, even though only a few **organic factors** seem to have a direct effect on the control of sexual desire.

Androgens such as testosterone appear to be necessary for a man's sexual desire. It appears that a minimum level of androgen is required for a man to be able to experience sexual desire. However, supra-physiological level of androgen in blood does not correlate with higher level of sexual desire.

Severe hyperprolactinaemia has a negative impact on sexual function, impairing sexual desire, as well as erectile function and testosterone production. A PRL-induced hypogonadism could explain, at least partially, this association. **Hypothyroidism** is another endocrine condition previously associated with male hypoactive sexual desire (HSD). The reasons for this association are unknown.

It is well known that psychiatric disorders, and in particular **major depression**, as well as their relative medical treatments, often induce a reduction of sexual desire. In addition, depression can freeze several aspects of a couple's sexual behaviour, which can be regarded as the cause or the consequence of a significant emotional distress. A longitudinal population study suggests that moderate or severe depression may cause erectile dysfunction (ED), and ED per se may cause or exacerbate depressive mood. On the other hand, psychological symptoms associated with depression, such as anhedonia, fatigue and low energy can affect sexual

Table 14.2 Drugs associated with male HSD

Antidepressants	Selective serotonin reuptake inhibitors (SSRIs)
	Tricyclic antidepressants
	Monoamine oxidase inhibitors
Antipsychotics	Typical
	Atypical
Lithium	
Antiepileptics	
Antiandrogens	GnRH analogues
	5α-reductase inhibitor
Clonidine	
Reserpine	
Opioids	

Source: Adapted from Corona and Maggi, 2012. Reproduced with permission from Medix.

functioning. Antidepressants can also affect libido, sexual arousal and orgasm/ejaculation. It is important to assess the role played by antidepressants in the sexual dysfunction of depressed patients (see Table 14.2).

A reduced male libido may also be present in many **chronic systemic diseases** such as kidney failure, chronic liver diseases, haematological diseases and HIV. In this case, the problem is multifactorial due to the presence of hormonal factors and intrapsychic and relational problems related to the deterioration of quality of life. Recently, it has been found that men with **prostatitis/chronic pelvic pain** syndrome reported significantly less frequent sexual desire or thoughts, less frequent sexual activities, less arousal/erectile function, less orgasm function and sexual pain than men without any pain condition.

HSDD has obvious consequences on sexual functioning. A decreased sexual motivation can result either in a decrease of sexual consumption and ED, or lower sexual activity and ED might result in a lower sexual desire. It is in this case that HSDD is probably an evasive reaction, put in place to reduce the anxiety related to the impaired sexual performance.

More in the case of **acquired/situational HSDD**, possible causes include intrapsychic problems (conflict in the couple, negative feelings), cognitive and cultural factors (sexual beliefs, automatic thoughts during sexual activity), intimacy difficulty, relationship troubles or other stressing life events.

Clinical evaluation

The detection of HSDD in men is not difficult if the clinician asks directly about desire, interest or wish for sexual activity. Most patients easily identify a change in their usual pattern and this is the way in which the condition is identified most of the time in clinical practice. Sometimes, it is necessary to investigate the indicators of sexual desire which, although not as direct as the expression of desire, could be a good clinical clue (see Table 14.3).

When a man presents himself with another sexual dysfunction, it is important to specifically look for the presence of HSDD. The management and eventual success of treatment depend on how the clinician effectively identifies and treats HSDD (see Box 14.1).

Table 14.3 Manifestations of sexual desire

Masturbation
Attempts to initiate sexual behaviour with a partner or receptivity to partner initiative
Erotic fantasies – daytime or nighttime thoughts about oneself in sexual interaction
Sexual attractions and responses to others
Spontaneous genital sensations of arousal accompanying erotic thoughts, identified as 'horniness' or 'randiness' by men, as sexual drive by clinicians

Source: Corona et al. 2013. Reproduced with permission from Medix.

Box 14.1 Questions to Diagnose HSDD and differentiate from another sexual dysfunction

To assess sexual desire (Always/Usually/Sometimes/Occasionally/Never):

Do you experience pleasurable thoughts about sex?
Do you initiate lovemaking?
Easy to get and stay aroused?
Sexual fantasies?
Responsive to partner's overture?
Self-stimulation?
Do you miss sex?

To investigate the problem:

Despite your lack of interest, can you still get an erection?
Compared to your past, how would you rate your interest in sex?
If you can get an erection, do you think you would be interested in having sex?
How frequent is your sexual activity? (if normal, ask if the activity is done without desire)
How often do you have thoughts about sex?
How often do you have sexual fantasies (do they include your partner?)
Who initiates sexual activity in your relationship and has it changed recently?

Source: Adapted from Corona et al. 2013. Reproduced with permission from Medix.

An example of a flowchart for the diagnosis of HSDD in men is reported in Figure 14.1.

An accurate medical history is the key point for the correct classification of the symptom HSDD. It is important to explore all the possible causes as well as substance abuse and use of medication. In generalized HSDD, physical examination (including examination of the genitals and signs of gynaecomastia or galactorrhoea) and endocrinological assessment (measurement of serum total testosterone, PRL and thyroid function) are needed. Please also see Chapter 10.

Treatment

Treatment of HSDD should be etiologically oriented. A comprehensive, integrative biopsychosocial approach to both the male's and the couple's sexuality is usually required.

When **hormonal disturbances** are detected, an adequate therapy might improve sexual desire even in the short term.

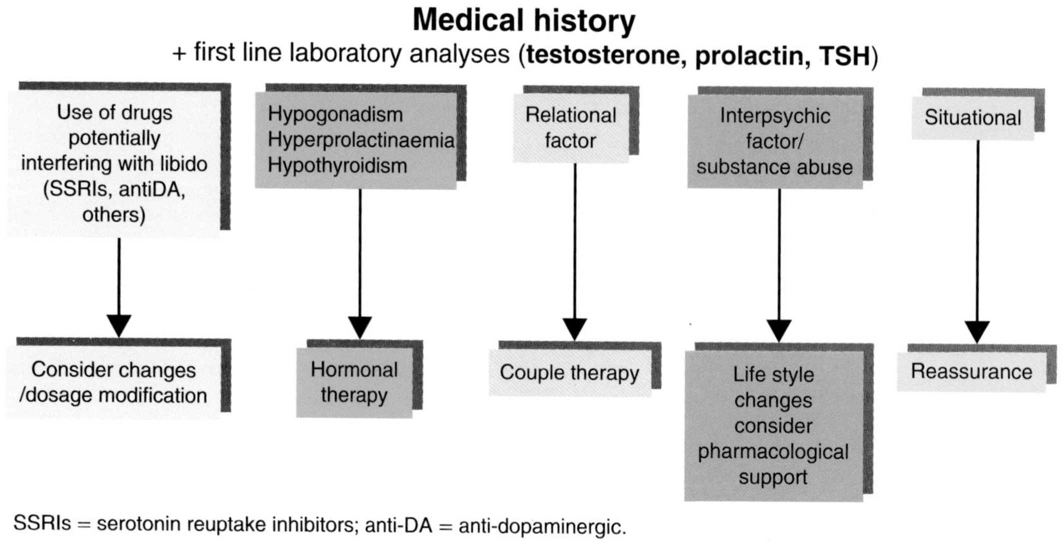

Medical history
+ first line laboratory analyses (testosterone, prolactin, TSH)

Use of drugs potentially interfering with libido (SSRIs, antiDA, others)	Hypogonadism Hyperprolactinaemia Hypothyroidism	Relational factor	Interpsychic factor/ substance abuse	Situational
↓	↓	↓	↓	↓
Consider changes /dosage modification	Hormonal therapy	Couple therapy	Life style changes consider pharmacological support	Reassurance

SSRIs = serotonin reuptake inhibitors; anti-DA = anti-dopaminergic.

Figure 14.1 Flow-chart for the diagnosis and treatment of HSDD. Source: Corona and Maggi, 2012. Reproduced with permission from Medix

In case of hyperprolactinaemia, the modification of the drug used is advisable. Dopamine-agonist agents are the first-choice treatment in case of pituitary secreting adenomas. Testosterone replacement therapy may be beneficial only in hypogonadal patients (total testosterone, (TT) < 12 nM). Thyroxin therapy is indicated in cases of hypothyroidism.

More complex is the situation due to **drugs potentially interfering with sexual desire**. The removal or the substitution of the drug are not always possible, even though it could resolve the problem. As mentioned above, HSD is a symptom of depression and antidepressants themselves can induce or worsen HSD. In these cases, the clinician should carefully evaluate the opportunity to change or adequately reduce current therapy.

When HSD is mainly supported by a disruption of the **relational or intrapsychic factors**, a short-term psychotherapy might be appropriate. Psychological approaches to low desire have a long history and have been found to be effective with sustained improvements over time.

The common aim is to encourage the recreational and hedonistic aspect of sexuality by exploring different erotic experiences. It is important to work on improving communication between partners, the lack of which is often at the bottom of the problem.

When conflict and relationship distress may cause low sexual desire, the patient and his partner should be referred to a couple/relationship therapy.

Currently, there is no **pharmaceutical approach** commercially available that can increase sexual desire.

Further reading

Brotto, L.A. & The, D.S.M. (2010) Diagnostic criteria for hypoactive sexual desire disorder in men. *Archives of Sexual Behaviour*, **7** (**6**), 2015–2030.

Carvalho, J. & Nobre, P. (2011) Biopsychosocial determinants of men's sexual desire: testing an integrative model. *The Journal of Sexual Medicine*, **8**, 754–763.

Corona, G. & Maggi, M. (2012) Hypoactive sexual desire (libido) disorder. In: Porst, H. & Reisman, Y. (eds), *ESSM Syllabus of Sexual Medicine*. Medix, Amsterdam.

Corona, G., Rastrelli, G., Ricca, V. *et al.* (2013) Risk factors associated with primary and secondary reduced libido in male patients with sexual dysfunction. *The Journal of Sexual Medicine*, **10**, 1074–1089.

Corona, G., Tripodi, F., Reisman, Y. & Maggi, M. (2013) Male hypoactive desire disorder. In: Kirana, P.S., Tripodi, F., Reisman, Y. & Porst, H. (eds), *EFS-ESSM Syllabus of Clinical Sexology*. Medix, Amsterdam.

DeRogatis, L., Rosen, R.C., Goldstein, I., Werneburg, B., Kempthorne-Rawson, J. & Sand, M. (2012) Characterization of hypoactive sexual desire disorder (HSDD) in men. *The Journal of Sexual Medicine*, **9**, 812–820.

Hackett, G.I. (2008) Disorders of male sexual desire. In: Rowland, D.L. & Incrocci, L. (eds), *Handbook of Sexual and Gender Identity Disorders*. John Wiley & Sons, Inc, Hoboken, NJ.

Levine, S.B. Hypoactive sexual desire disorder in men: basic types, causes, and treatment. *Psychiatric Times*, 2010, pp.40–43.

Meuleman, E.J. & Van Lankveld, J. (2005) Hypoactive sexual desire disorder: an underestimated condition in men. *BJU International*, **95**, 201–296.

Rubio-Aurioles, E. & Bivalacqua, T.J. (2013) Standard operational procedures for low sexual desire in men. *The Journal of Sexual Medicine*, **10**, 94–107.

CHAPTER 15

Problems of Sexual Desire and Arousal in Women

Lori A. Brotto[1] and Ellen T.M. Laan[2]

[1]University of British Columbia, Vancouver, Canada
[2]Academic Medical Centre, University of Amsterdam, Amsterdam, The Netherlands

---

> **OVERVIEW**
>
> - Problems with sexual desire and sexual arousal are no longer considered to be separate sexual problems
> - Sexual desire/arousal results from an interplay of a sensitive sexual response system and effective stimuli that activate this system
> - In the context of a sexual relationship, problems that are presented as a lack, or loss, of sexual desire can usually be reframed as differences in sexual desire and in differences in what kind of sex is desired
> - A biopsychosocial sexual history from a longitudinal perspective is mandatory for making the diagnosis
> - Because most problems become manifest in, are associated with, or are caused by the relational context, the partner needs to be involved in assessment and treatment
> - Enhancing sexual pleasure of both partners is a crucial factor in long-lasting improvement of the sexual relationship

Introduction

A distressing lack of interest in sexual activity that persists is the most common reason why women seek sex therapy. Early studies show that at least one-third of women younger than 59 reported low sexual desire over the past year. Because less than 28% of sexual difficulties (defined as being present for 1 month) persist for 6 months or more, only enduring and distressing symptoms should be considered representative of a desire disorder. When one takes into account the presence of clinically significant distress associated with low sexual desire, the prevalence drops to approximately 8–12%. Multinational studies have found higher rates of low sexual interest in Middle East and Southeast Asian countries, emphasizing the importance of cultural sensitivity when assessing sexual interest and arousal (see Table 15.1). There is considerable research interest in women's low sexual desire and this is amplified by the fact that, to date, there are no Federal Drug Administration (FDA)-approved pharmaceutical treatments available contributing to an aggressive (and expensive) race to find the panacea unlocking women's lost sexual desire.

ABC of Sexual Health, Third Edition. Edited by Kevan Wylie.
© 2015 John Wiley & Sons, Ltd. Published 2015 by John Wiley & Sons, Ltd.

Original conceptualizations of sexual desire framed it as an intrinsic part of the human experience, emerging from internal drive states much like hunger or thirst. This view contributed to a linear, tri-phasic model of sexual response in which it was believed that sexual desire was the initiator of a sequence of phases leading to arousal and subsequently orgasm. More recent conceptualizations, however, frame sexual desire as emerging from the experience of sexual arousal. The Incentive Motivation Model proposes that sexual desire directly emerges from, and is difficult to separate from, sexual arousal. In this view, feelings of sexual arousal and desire are both responses to a sexually relevant stimulus. They may be phenomenologically distinguished in that feelings of sexual arousal may represent the awareness of genital changes resulting from sexual stimulation, perhaps combined with a conscious evaluation that the situation is indeed 'sexual', whereas feelings of desire may represent the experience of a willingness to behave in a sexual way.

To date, problems with sexual desire and sexual arousal are no longer considered to be separate sexual problems. In the fifth edition of the Diagnostic and Statistical Manual of Mental Disorders (DSM-5, 2013), such problems are classified as 'Sexual Interest/Arousal Disorder' (SIAD). Unlike previous definitions of hypoactive sexual desire disorder (HSDD), SIAD is based on polythetic criteria, which recognizes that sexual desire and arousal may be experienced differently across different women.

Aetiology

Sexual desire/arousal is inherently a biopsychosocial experience. Therefore, in cases of low or absent desire/arousal, the clinician should consider the biological, psychological, sexual and socio-cultural influences associated with the change in desire/arousal, and the ongoing factors sustaining the difficulty. A longitudinal perspective in which the clinician considers the predisposing factors (i.e. the events predating the sexual difficulty that may have made a woman vulnerable to developing low desire/arousal), the precipitating factors (i.e. those occurring in temporal proximity to the onset of dysfunction), and the perpetuating factors (i.e. the current events/factors that maintain the problem of low desire) allows for a comprehensive view of the chronology of the problem. It is also important for the clinician to consider the 'protective' factors (i.e. those aspects of the woman's self or relationship or context that mitigate some of the negative influences on her desire).

Table 15.1 Prevalence of low sexual desire in women

Study	Sample characteristics	Prevalence
Laumann et al. (1999)	1,749 partnered, American women aged 18–59	27–32% low desire (distress not assessed)
Fugl-Meyer and Sjogren Fugl-Meyer (1999)	1,335 Swedish women aged 18–74	34% had low desire (defined as often/nearly all the time/all the time). Amongst these, 43% viewed it as a problem
Mercer et al. (2003)	11,161 British men and women aged 16-44	40% had low desire for at least 1 month; 10% had low desire for at least 6 months
Bancroft et al. (2003)	987 American women aged 20–65	7.2% prevalence of low desire
Oberg et al. (2004)	1,056 Swedish women aged 19–65	60% mild low desire, 29% manifest low desire
Laumann et al. (2005)	9,000 sexually active multinational women aged 40–80	26–43%
Leiblum et al. (2006)	952 sexually active American surgically or naturally postmenopausal women aged 20–70	24–36% had low desire. Rates of HSDD ranged from 9% to 26%
Dennerstein et al. (2006)	2,467 sexually active European women aged 20–70	16–46%. Rates of HSDD ranged from 7% to 16%
Witting et al. (2008)	5,463 Finnish women aged 18–49	Using a FSFI cut-off score of 3.16, 55% had low desire. Using a FSDS cut-off score of 8.75, 23% had low desire and distress
Shifren et al. (2008)	13,581 American women aged 18–102	34% had low desire, overall 10% had low desire and distress
Mitchell et al. (2009)	6,942 British women aged 16–44	10.7% reported lack of desire for 6 months or more. 27.9% of those sought help

FSDS: Female sexual distress scale.
FSFI: Female sexual function index.
HSDD: Hypoactive sexual desire disorder.

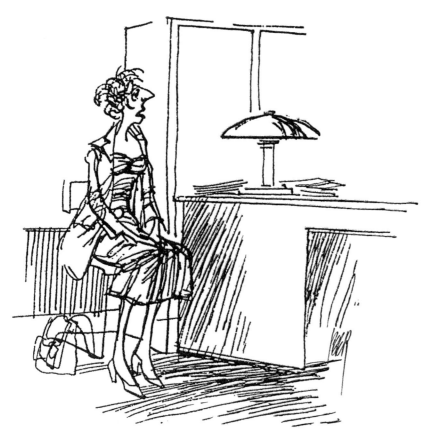

"MY HUSBAND AND I HAVE A LOUSY SEX LIFE, BUT HE DOESN'T KNOW THAT."

Figure 15.1 Particularly in women, sexual desire/arousal seems to be sensitive to the interpersonal aspects of the relationship. Source: © Peter van Straaten, reproduced with permission

Particularly in women, sexual desire/arousal seems to be sensitive to the interpersonal aspects of the relationship. Being in a relationship characterized by healthy and open communication can be a protective factor that is capitalized on in therapy (Figure 15.1).

The Incentive Motivation Model is one that provides a succinct method for conceptualizing sexual desire/arousal in women. It posits that sexual desire/arousal results from an interplay of a sensitive sexual response system and effective stimuli that activate this system. The sensitivity of the sexual response system is determined by biological factors (hormones and neurotransmitters) as well as (conditioned) expectations based on past experiences. Compared to former linear models of sexual response, which predicted that sexual desire was the initiator of a sexual response system, and that desire triggered arousal and orgasm in linear sequence, more contemporary models emphasize the circular nature of sexual response and highlight the important role of internal and external stimuli that trigger desire for sex. Within such a framework, sexual desire and sexual arousal are seen as simultaneous responses to a sexually relevant stimulus (i.e. a stimulus that the individual perceives as being sufficiently sexual). Stimuli are given high priority, but may only elicit sexual response if activated in a reactive system that allows for sexual responsiveness. Because biological as well as psychological factors can influence the responsiveness of the sexual system and the effectiveness of sexual stimuli to elicit sexual response, an evaluation of biological, psychological and sociocultural influences must form a part of a thorough assessment of SIAD.

Assessment

Clinicians may find the assessment/treatment algorithm presented in Figure 15.2 to be useful. The assessment of women with sexual desire and arousal problems is based on a structured interview, physical examination and to a limited degree, laboratory investigation. The clinician should inquire about both frequency and intensity of sexual interest, fantasies/erotic thoughts, pleasure during sex and physical (including genital and non-genital) sensations. Each of the domains outlined in Table 15.2 should be assessed using a face-to-face interview format. Within this structured interview, the clinician should fully assess the presenting problem including its history, type of onset and whether it is generalized or situational. There should also be a medical history as well as psychological/psychiatric history taking. Developmental history, including family of origin themes, along with a past sexual history (including any presence of sexual abuse or harassment) are also useful components of a comprehensive interview.

Comprehensive sexual interview

Assessment using the Incentive Motivation Model requires a detailed assessment of past and current sexual activities. A woman's disinterest may well be directly related to the sexual activity that usually takes place. Detailed probing of the kind of sexual activity that she would desire may reveal that her sexual desire is stimulus- and context-dependent. Many clinicians may shy away from such a detailed assessment, for fear of invading an individual's or a

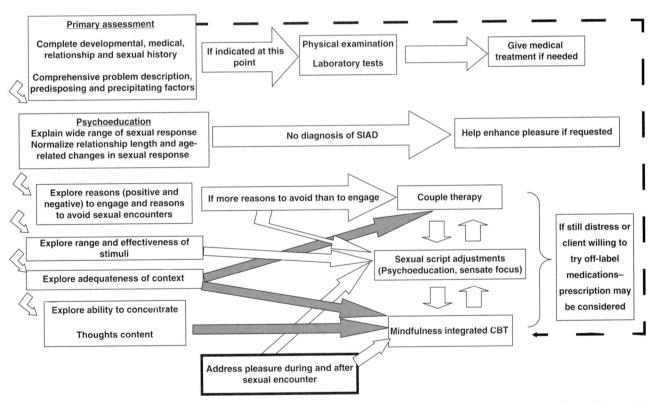

Figure 15.2 Treatment diagram to illustrate the recommended steps for intervention. After initial assessment, if medical problems are found, further medical examination and treatment are warranted. If psychological or couple issues are first detected, client may benefit from treatment focusing on cognitive processing, mindfulness skills and behavioural changes. In some cases, couple therapy is needed. Psychoeducation is imperative to overcome unfavourable beliefs and to define and adjust expectations. If there are little or no motivations to be sexual, sexual stimuli are not satisfactory, thoughts content is distracting or disturbing, mindfulness integrated CBT is recommended. Address sexual scripts and develop alternatives as needed. Address pleasure. Off-label medications are indicated only if previous steps were unsuccessful, after the client received full explanation on the limitations of medical treatment. Source: Binik and Hall (2007), Reprinted with permission by Guilford Press

Table 15.2 Domains to assess for women presenting with sexual desire/arousal concerns

Biological	Hormones	Steroid hormones activate mechanisms of sexual excitation by directing the synthesis of enzymes and receptors for several neurochemical systems. Serum oestradiol associated with vulvar-vaginal atrophy, but not consistently associated with desire. The relationship between serum testosterone and women's sexual desire is equivocal, with some studies showing a significant relationship and others showing no relationship. Clinically available assays lack accuracy in measuring serum testosterone in women. Neurosteroids thought to play a role in sexual desire but direct measurement is not possible. Some evidence that synthetic progestins may have negative effects on sexual desire
	Neurotransmitters	Dopamine is a major neurotransmitter involved in sexual arousal due to its actions in mesolimbic and hypothalamic circuits
	Medical conditions	Medical conditions affecting the circulatory, endocrine, musculoskeletal and central nervous systems are important to take into account in the presence of sexual interest and arousal complaints
	Medications	Prescription and recreational drugs/substances have myriad effects on sexual response and should be assessed
Relational	Relationship-related	A woman's feelings for her partner are a major determinant of her sexual desire. Emotional intimacy is often a predictor of desire; however, as emotional intimacy increases with relationship duration, there may be a negative effect on sexual desire. In married women, feelings of institutionalization of the relationship, over-familiarity and de-sexualization of roles can dampen sexual desire. A clinician must therefore balance concerns about a woman's complaints of loss of motivation for once highly passionate and erotic sex in the context of a long-term relationship
	Partner-related	A partner's sexual functioning can impact women's motivation for sex. For example, premature ejaculation in men is often comorbid with low sexual desire in women. Poor sexual technique or particularly rigid sexual beliefs about sexual technique; sexual needs that the woman believes she cannot satisfy; and a partner to whom the woman is not attracted all impact desire
Individual	Mood	Mood instability, low self-esteem, and having an introverted personality style are associated with decreased sexual interest and may all influence the responsivity of the sexual system. Depression significantly increases the odds of having low sexual interest by at least twofold amongst women aged 40–80, and loss of sexual desire is common in major depressive disorder
	Anxiety	Cognitive distraction during sexual activity negatively impacts women's sexual esteem, sexual arousal, sexual satisfaction and orgasm consistency. Sexual satisfaction in particular was influenced by distracting thoughts while being sexual with a partner. Anxiety itself has a negative impact on sexual motivation and arousal
Sociocultural factors	Lack of sexual knowledge	Knowledge about what sexual activities and sexual positions are best suitable to generate sexual pleasure and orgasm in women may be an important factor in a woman's loss of sexual desire/arousal. A strong focus on sexual intercourse as the goal of any sexual interaction may be a major disadvantage in her ability to gain sexual rewards
	Negative media messages	Negative messages about masturbation in girls and the view of women as passive recipients of men's sexual desires and actions may encourage a passive attitude to sexual activity and inhibit women's sexual interest. Failure to meet cultural norms concerning sexual attractiveness or sexual response, conflict between the sexual norms of culture of origin and those of the dominant culture, may trigger loss of motivation for sex
	Fatigue	Personal and family stressors, lack of sleep, competing demands
	Culture/ethnicity	There are marked cross-cultural differences in the prevalence of desire difficulties, and in the view of sexual activity as procreative versus recreative. Culture-linked differences in sex guilt also impact upon desire

couple's personal space or of being seen as voyeuristic. However, without detailed knowledge about what kinds of sexual activities are taking place and the extent to which these activities generate sexual feelings, it is simply not possible to provide adequate help. An additional advantage of such an assessment is that it sends the message that talking about sex is not only ok, but essential for sexual health. Owing to the fact that sexual functioning in women is strongly influenced by relational context, it is of great importance to talk to both the woman and her partner; preferably, the couple is seen together. Questions may be asked with respect to (variety in) types of sexual activities (solo and partnered), use of imagery (sexual fantasy), use of (additional) tactile (e.g. vibratory) and visual stimulation, and the conditions in which sexual activity takes place (Box 15.1).

> **Box 15.1 Questions to ask in a comprehensive sexual interview**
>
> - To what extent is she aware of genital response during sexual stimulation?
> - How does she value sexual stimulation, and what, if anything, is responsible for a change in how sexual stimulation is appreciated over the years?
> - What does she do when the stimulation provided is (no longer) pleasurable? Does she feel free to suggest alternative modes of stimulation or is she assuming that she 'should' feel pleasure by what is provided and that the fact that she does not, must mean that there is something wrong with her?

- Is she aware of the fact that the extent to which direct glans clitoris stimulation is pleasurable may depend on her level of arousal and may therefore change over the course of lovemaking?
- Is she trying to tolerate genital stimulation that is not or no longer pleasurable because she feels that suggestions for alternatives may disappoint the partner or may be perceived as criticism?
- Is she and/or is her partner expecting her to become sexually aroused and be orgasmic by sexual intercourse alone?
- Does she perhaps actively avoid sexual stimuli in one way or another, because they are not (or no longer) acceptable or pleasant to her (or her partner)? For example, is she avoiding intimate physical contact for fear that her partner will then expect to have sexual intercourse?
- Is sexual intercourse painful? If so, why would she require of herself to desire something that is painful?
- Is the couple aware of the fact that in both sexes, sexual arousal usually requires longer and more direct genital stimulation as both age?
- Is she able to experience orgasm?
- Can the woman allow herself to stay relaxed and focused during sexual stimulation?
- She may know what she does not desire sexually, but does she know what (kinds of touching or sexual activities) she would desire?
- If not, would she be willing to open herself up to sexual touch and to explore what might entice her sexually?
- Would her partner be willing to help her to explore her sexual possibilities if she prefers this to be done in a partnered context?

Contextual factors

A detailed assessment of contextual factors that influence sexual response is also essential. These would include variables in the environment (e.g. privacy, environmental distractions), in the relationship (e.g. emotional sharing and intimacy, feelings for partner, attraction to partner, a partner's own sexual dysfunction) and in the woman herself (e.g. her appraisal of her own physical and genital attractiveness, a history of negative sexual experiences/pain/abuse, mood, worries/anxiety, medications, medical comorbidities that negatively affect sexual response). It is this combination of positive incentives, appropriate stimuli and a context conducive to sexual response that sets the stage for sexual arousal and desire – a desire for the sexual activity to continue for now more sexual reasons, in addition to whatever initial incentives were present. If the outcome is rewarding (emotionally and physically), she might have more motivation to initiate or respond to cues in the future.

Medical history and physical and laboratory evaluations

Various medical diseases involving the autonomic nervous and vascular system are known risk factors for problems with sexual desire/arousal (Giraldi *et al.*, 2013). These include diabetes, neurological disorders such as multiple sclerosis and spinal cord

injuries. Other medical conditions may also indirectly affect sexual desire/arousal if the treatment of these conditions includes surgeries on the pelvis and the genitals. Medications such as serotonin re-uptake inhibitors (SSRIs), antipsychotics, mood stabilizers, cardiovascular medications, chemotherapy agents and hypertension drugs may affect sexual response, although factors associated with the reasons for taking the medications (e.g. nerve damage, anxiety, depression) are often hard to distinguish from the actual effects of the medication.

A physical examination is rarely used to make a diagnosis of SIAD. However, it can be very useful for providing education around vulvar anatomy and physiology. In cases of sexual pain, vulvovaginal atrophy related to menopause, breastfeeding, treatment with low-oestrogen or progesterone-only contraceptives, and in hypothalamic or pituitary disease, a physical examination can identify the contributors to a reduced genital response. Laboratory evaluations are rarely of use in the diagnosis of women's desire and arousal problems. Oestrogen deficiency is best detected by history and a physical examination. Serum androgen levels do not correlate with sexual function and are currently not recommended (Brotto *et al.*, 2010). It should be noted though that research in this area is hindered by a lack of standardized assays suitable for detecting androgens in the female range. Please also see Chapter 10.

Diagnosis

A diagnosis of SIAD requires any three of the following six criteria: (i) absent/reduced interest in sexual activity; (ii) absent/reduced sexual/erotic thoughts or fantasies; (iii) No/reduced initiation of sexual activity, and typically unreceptive to a partner's attempts to initiate; (iv) absent/reduced sexual excitement/pleasure during sexual activity on almost all or all (approximately 75–100%) sexual encounters; (v) absent/reduced sexual interest/arousal in response to any internal or external sexual/erotic cues (e.g. written, verbal, visual) and (vi) Absent/reduced genital and/or non-genital sensations during sexual activity on almost all or all (approx. 75–100%) sexual encounters (in identified situational contexts or, if generalized, in all contexts). The difficulties must persist for a minimum of approximately 6 months, and create clinically significant distress. Single women seldomly present with the complaint of low or absent sexual desire/arousal. Usually the complaint is presented by women in a steady relationship, and distress associated with the difficulties is often related to differences in sexual desire between partners. DSM-5 explicitly states that a desire discrepancy between partners is not sufficient to diagnose SIAD in the low desire/arousal partner. There are no objective criteria, however, to establish how much disinterest is required in order to qualify for a SIAD diagnosis.

The following two clinical scenarios illustrate how the SIAD criteria allow for different expressions of low sexual desire/arousal across women.

Clinical Scenario 1

Barbara presents for sex therapy with the primary complaint of 'I don't feel any sexual excitement any longer'. Upon probing, she reveals that she rarely thinks about sex with her partner, although she continues to have sexual intercourse on a weekly basis. She does not initiate sexual activity, and she only very reluctantly accepts her partner's sexual solicitations for fear of losing the relationship. Sexual touching elicits few, if any, positive sexual sensations, and she is minimally aware of vaginal lubrication. On most occasions of sexual activity, the encounter ends with her feeling physically and emotionally dissatisfied; however, on a few occasions she is able to become sexually aroused in her mind to a limited degree. These problems have existed for the past 5 years and have led Barbara to withdraw emotionally from her 15-year relationship. She avoids physical contact as much as possible, for fear that it will lead to a sexual overture from her partner.

Clinical Scenario 2

Veronika (age 32, married) experienced frequent sexual desire and a very robust sexual arousal response with her husband until the birth of her child when she experienced a marked decline in the frequency of sexual desire. She continues, however, to become sexually aroused and orgasmic during sexual activity, particularly if she is well-rested, and this triggers responsive desire during the encounter.

The 6-month criterion rules out adaptive changes in sexual desire that may be related to transient events in a woman's life (e.g. stressor, medical illness, fatigue). The clinician must inquire about both the frequency and intensity of sexual interest, fantasies/erotic thoughts, pleasure during sex, and physical sensations. Women with acquired low desire have a more restricted range of effective stimuli that elicit sexual interest and arousal (McCall and Meston, 2006), and appraise sexual stimuli in a less positive way (both consciously and automatically) than women without sexual problems (Brauer *et al.*, 2012). This finding underscores the necessity of exploring the range of sexual stimuli that might elicit the woman's sexual interest and arousal, along with her current and past response to such stimuli. The assessment of clinically significant distress is a key aspect of making the diagnosis of SIAD. Distress is often what prompts treatment seeking. When one considers distress, the prevalence of a desire dysfunction drops considerably compared to the much more common prevalence of non-distressing symptoms of low desire. The clinician will note that clinically significant distress must be experienced *in the individual*; however, a partner's distress may often be the elicitor of treatment-seeking. In cases of loss of sexual desire due to severe relationship discord, a diagnosis of SIAD is not made.

Treatment

Education

Knowledge about what sexual activities and sexual positions are best suitable to generate sexual pleasure and orgasm in women may be an important factor in helping a woman with her problems of sexual desire/arousal. A strong focus on sexual intercourse as the goal of any sexual interaction may be a major disadvantage in her ability to gain sexual rewards (sexual pleasure and orgasm), as data show that intercourse without additional glans clitoris stimulation results in orgasm in only about 25–30% of heterosexual women (Lloyd, 2005). This contrasts sharply with research suggesting that over 90% of heterosexual men always orgasm during sexual

intercourse (Douglass and Douglass, 1997). This is not explained by women simply being less able to orgasm, as women who have sex with women orgasm in about 80% of all sexual interactions (de Bruijn, 1982). Education should enhance awareness of the fact that for women, in contrast to men, sexual intercourse alone is a relatively ineffective means of sexual stimulation. She should not regard herself as abnormal if she does not experience much sexual pleasure from sexual intercourse alone, or if she cannot experience orgasm with this activity. The inability to experience orgasm during intercourse in the absence of additional glans clitoris stimulation is now considered a 'normal variation of sexual response' rather than a 'pathological inhibition'. At the beginning of the twentieth century Freud wrote that women who required glans clitoral stimulation for orgasm are psychologically 'immature' and that mature women would be able to have a 'vaginal orgasm' (i.e. an orgasm by means of intercourse only, not involving the clitoris), a view that is held by some even today (Brody and Costa, 2008). Education about the anatomy of the clitoris may reveal that it is hard to imagine any type of sexual activity, including vaginal intercourse, that does not involve the clitoris. The visible button-like portion of the clitoris (the glans) is located near the front junction of the labia minora (inner lips), above the opening of the urethra. A much larger part of the clitoris, not visible from the outside, forms a wishbone-shaped structure containing the corpora cavernosa and vestibular bulbs and may extend into the vagina's anterior wall (see Figure 15.3). The glans, and to a greater extent the clitoral body, swell up during sexual stimulation and are the main source of sexual pleasure. If one understands the anatomy of the clitoris one understands that unaroused intercourse, that is intercourse without adequate 'foreplay' that is sexually arousing, will not generate sexual pleasure and orgasm. In many cases, it may even be an important cause of dyspareunia.

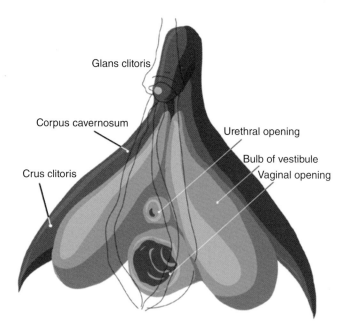

Figure 15.3 The internal anatomy of the human vulva, with the clitoral hood and labia minora indicated as lines. The clitoris extends from the visible portion to a point below the pubic bone. (Accessed at http://en.wikipedia.org/wiki/File:Clitoris_anatomy_labeled-en.svg). Picture released to the public domain

Many women may find that education and opportunity for discussion with an empathic and informative clinician is sufficient for arming them to make improvements in their sexual lives and desire. For other women and their partners, a more rigorous approach is needed. In this case, referral to either a licensed sex therapist and/or a psychotherapist specialized in relationship problems may be warranted.

Psycho(sexual) Therapy

Psychosexual treatment formats are aimed at helping the woman and her partner to employ (new) sexual stimuli that can lead to arousal, strengthening the rewarding value of sex by promoting pleasant sexual feelings, decreasing any negative feelings concerning sexuality and the partner, and optimizing communication and intimacy within the relationship. Although evidence for its effectiveness is lacking, sensate focus exercises developed in the 1970s by Masters and Johnson, aimed at enhancing sexual arousal and orgasmic function, are part of the standard repertoire in most psychosexual treatments. In order for sexual desire/arousal to occur and to allow it to build, one needs to be open to sexual stimulation, be unafraid to 'let go' and, to some extent, 'lose control'. In a sexual relationship, there is the additional need to feel sufficiently safe to allow these things to happen in front of another person.

The literature evaluating psychosexual treatments is sparse. Two treatments that have received attention, cognitive behavioural therapy (CBT) and mindfulness-based interventions (MBIs), involve interventions aimed at enhancing sensitivity to sexual stimulation. CBT is a change-oriented approach that involves identifying and challenging problematic beliefs that give rise to sex-related avoidance and negative emotions. MBIs, on the other hand, are acceptance-based, and involve a system of cultivating present-moment, nonjudgmental awareness, without any deliberate attempt to change one's experience. At present, we can conclude that there is promising evidence for these methods in improving women's low desire and arousal, but much more research is needed (Table 15.3).

Medications

Pharmacological treatments have been of immense interest and the focus of many empirical studies since the approval of sildenafil citrate in the late 1990s. However, despite extensive research on a variety of topical and oral agents, there are no FDA-approved medications to ameliorate women's complaints of loss of desire and arousal. In the UK, postmenopausal women with distressing low sexual desire may be a candidate for testosterone therapy if biomedical and psychosocial causes of her low desire have been ruled out (British Society for Sexual Medicine, 2010). In 2005, a transdermal form of testosterone became available in Europe for women with bilateral oophorectomy plus hysterectomy who are also receiving oestrogens. Remarkably, the testosterone patch was removed from the European market in 2012 for commercial reasons. Tibolone, a pharmaceutical with oestrogenic, progestogenic as well as androgenic characteristics and registered in Europe for hormone supplementation therapy in postmenopausal women with oestrogen deficiency complaints, has more positive effect on

Table 15.3 Psychological treatments for women's sexual desire/arousal difficulties

Type of treatment	Treatment components	Outcomes
CBT – individual	Eight weeks that includes sensate focus, directed masturbation, and the coital alignment technique	Significant improvements in sexual desire with lasting gains 6 months later
CBT – group	Twelve weeks	Significant reductions in HSDD severity with sustained gains even a year after treatment
Mindfulness – group	Three monthly sessions that included in-session mindfulness practice as well as daily at-home practice, along with sex education, and cognitive therapy	Significant improvements in sexual desire, sex-related distress and perceptions of genital tingling amongst women with HSDD
Mindfulness – group	Two biweekly sessions that involved exclusive practice of mindfulness meditation	Amongst women with sex-related distress associated with a history of sexual abuse, there were significant improvements in sexual functioning and in genital sexual arousal

various aspects of sexual functioning and psychological well-being than oestrogen therapy alone. Table 15.4 provides a summary of the various tested pharmaceutical agents, their mode of action, and their efficacy.

The placebo response in studies of pharmaceutical products designed to improve women's sexual desire is marked, with most studies showing at least a 40% efficacy in placebo arms. A consideration of the placebo response, defined as a substance/procedure administered with the hope of improving symptoms but which contains no active therapeutic ingredients (unknown to the recipient), is important as it may tell the clinician important information about the mechanisms of change. The placebo response is affected by the conditions that surround treatment, such as discussion with an attentive and empathic care provider, the sense of normalization that accompanies discussing a problem, and so on. Table 15.5 considers the various ways in which a placebo response may improve sexual function in women.

In the future, more pharmacological treatments may enter the market for women with sexual problems. However, it should be noted that pharmacological facilitation of sexual arousal will only be successful when the treatment also focuses on psychological and relational factors. When a woman has predominantly negative or very little rewarding sexual experience, there will be very few stimuli that can elicit feelings of arousal. Furthermore, in a predominantly negative relational context, the woman will be reluctant to respond to sexual stimulation. Therefore, stimulation of sexual arousal with medication alone cannot be expected to be very effective (Laan and Both, 2011).

Table 15.4 Medications that have been the focus of empirical research for improving women's sexual desire/arousal

Agent	Mode of delivery	Efficacy	Availability
Oestrogen	Tablets, pessaries/vagitories, cream, vaginal ring	Current standard of care for treatment of vulvovaginal atrophy. If low desire is secondary to this, then desire may improve	Approved by FDA
Testosterone	Patch	Naturally and surgically menopausal oestrogen-replete and non-replete women who reported a decline in their desire for sex have found a benefit of a 300 μg/day testosterone patch	Off-label use only in the USA but approved by the European Medicines Agency. Concerns about the high rate of androgenic side effects (30% of women) and concerns about long-term safety remain
Tibolone (a selective tissue oestrogenic activity regulator)	Oral	Tibolone has shown increases in sexual desire, frequency of arousability, sexual fantasies and vaginal lubrication versus placebo	Available in 90 countries but not in North America. Some concern about the risk of recurrence of breast cancer and the risk of stroke in older women (60–85 years)
DHEA (converts into androgens as well as oestrogens, possibly exerting benefits on all three layers of the vaginal wall)	Topical	Vaginal application of DHEA for postmenopausal vaginal atrophy significantly improves sexual desire/interest, sexual arousal, orgasm and pain	Off-label use
Buproprion (a noradrenaline and dopamine reuptake inhibitor)	Oral	In women with SSRI-associated mixed sexual symptoms, 4 weeks of treatment led to a significant increase in self-reported feelings of desire and sexual activity	Off-label use
Bremelanotide (an alpha-melanocyte-stimulating hormone analogue)	Subcutaneous	—	Undergoing clinical trials
Apomorphine (dopaminergic agent)	Oral	Significantly improved sexual function in women with HSDD. Side-effects were mainly nausea, vomiting and dizziness	Not available
Flibanserin (a 5-hydroxytryptophan (HT) 1A receptor agonist, 5-HT 2A receptor antagonist and dopamine D4 receptor partial agonist)	Oral	Premenopausal women with HSDD had significant improvements in sexually satisfying events with daily treatment of 100 mg flibanserin (but not 25 or 50 mg), and in sex-related distress and total sexual function. No effect on desire measured with a daily diary. 10% experienced side-effects of somnolence, dizziness and nausea	Not available
Sildenafil citrate (a phosphodiesterase type-5 inhibitor)	Oral	Women with anorgasmia associated with SSRI use had significant reversal of symptoms following the addition of sildenafil citrate (50 or 100 mg)	Off-label use
Lybrido (0.5 mg testosterone in a cyclodextrin carrier combined with 50 mg sildenafil citrate in a powder-filled gelatin capsule)	Oral	Only amongst women with low desire due to relatively insensitive system for sexual cues (n = 29): higher genital arousal response to a fantasy (but not to sexual films) compared to placebo; significantly higher sexual satisfaction during sexual events; significantly higher monthly reports of desire (but not weekly) compared to placebo. Lybrido had no effect on women with low desire who were highly sensitive to sexual cues	Undergoing Phase III clinical trials
Lybridos (0.5 mg testosterone in a cyclodextrin carrier combined with 10 mg buspirone in a powder-filled gelatin capsule)	Oral	Amongst women who were considered to be 'high inhibitors' (i.e. those with high acute serotonergic inhibitory control) (n = 28), treatment yielded significantly higher genital arousal response to a fantasy (but not to sexual films) as well as subjective reports of desire compared to placebo; significantly higher sexual satisfaction during sexual events; significantly higher weekly and monthly reports of desire compared to placebo. Lybridos had no effect on women with low desire and who had low inhibitory mechanisms	Undergoing clinical trials

HT: Hydroxytryptophan.
DHEA: Dehydroepiandrostenedione.

Table 15.5 Possible mechanisms by which the placebo response improves women's sexual function

Procedural aspects	Behavioural change associated with participating in a clinical trial (e.g. increased attention to one's sexuality, journaling). Increase in sexual frequency as a method of testing whether the medication 'worked'. Interaction with an interested investigator/clinician
Expectancies	Individual who believes they have received active treatment may interpret subsequent behaviours/experiences as being the result of taking an effective medication. Recipient may interpret 'side effects' as an indication of therapeutic efficacy
Partner reactions	Women's partners may exert subtle influence on a woman's desire through their expectations that the woman received an active treatment'

Acknowledgements

The authors thank the many women who generously shared their personal stories of sexual interest and arousal, and associated loss.

Further reading

American Psychiatric Association (2013) *Diagnostic and Statistical Manual of Mental Disorders*, 5th edn. American Psychiatric Association, Washington, DC.

Bancroft, J., Loftus, J. & Long, J.S. (2003) Distress about sex: a national survey of women in heterosexual relationships. *Archives of Sexual Behavior*, **32**, 193–208.

Basson, R. (2001a) Human sex-response cycles. *Journal of Sex & Marital Therapy*, **27**, 33–43.

Basson, R. (2001b) Using a different model for female sexual response to address women's problematic low sexual desire. *Journal of Sex & Marital Therapy*, **27**, 395–403.

Binik, Y.M. & Hall, K.S.K. (2007) *Principles and Practice of Sex Therapy*, 4th edn. Guildford Press.

Bradford, A. (2013) Listening to placebo in clinical trials for female sexual dysfunction. *Journal of Sexual Medicine*, **10**, 451–459.

Brauer, M., van Leeuwen, M., Janssen, E., Newhouse, S.K., Heiman, J.R. & Laan, E. (2012) Attentional and affective processing of sexual stimuli in women with hypoactive desire disorder. *Archives of Sexual Behavior*, **41**, 891–905.

British Society for Sexual Medicine (2010) Guidelines on the management of sexual problems in women: The role of androgens, http://www.bssm.org.uk/downloads/UK_Guidelines_Androgens_Female_2010.pdf (accessed 20 November 2014).

Brody, S. & Costa, R.M. (2008) Vaginal orgasm is associated with less use of immature psychological defense mechanisms. *Journal of Sexual Medicine*, **5**, 1167–1176.

Brotto, L.A., Bitzer, J., Laan, E., Leiblum, S. & Luria, M. (2010) Summary of the recommendations from committee 24: women's sexual desire and arousal disorders. *Journal of Sexual Medicine*, **7**, 586–614.

de Bruijn, G. (1982) From masturbation to orgasm with a partner: how some women bridge the gap – and why others don't. *Journal of Sex and Marital Therapy*, **8**, 151–167.

Dennerstein, L., Koochaki, P., Barton, I. & Graziottin, A. (2006) Hypoactive sexual desire disorder in menopausal women: a survey of Western European women. *Journal of Sexual Medicine*, **3**, 212–222.

Douglass, M. & Douglass, L. (1997) *Are We Having Fun Yet?* Hyperion, New York.

Everaerd, W. & Laan, E. (1995) Desire for passion: energetics of sexual response. *Journal of Sex & Marital Therapy*, **21**, 255–263.

Fugl-Meyer, A.R. & Sjogren Fugl-Meyer, K. (1999) Sexual disabilities, problems and satisfaction in 18–74 year old Swedes. *Scandinavian Journal of Sexology*, **2**, 79–105.

Giraldi, A., Rellini, A.H. & Laan, E. (2013) Standard operating procedures for female sexual arousal disorder: consensus of the International Society for Sexual Medicine. *Journal of Sexual Medicine*, **10**, 58–73.

Hayes, R.D., Bennett, C.M., Fairley, C.K. & Dennerstein, L. (2006) What can prevalence studies tell us about female sexual difficulty and dysfunction? *Journal of Sexual Medicine*, **3**, 589–595.

Kaplan, H.S. (1979) *Disorders of Sexual Desire*. Brunner/Mazel, New York.

Laan, E. & Both, S. (2008) What makes women experience desire? *Feminism and Psychology*, **18**, 505–514.

Laan, E. & Both, S. (2011) Sexual desire and arousal disorders in women. In: Balon, R. (ed), *Sexual Dysfunction: Beyond the Brain-Body Connection*. Advances in Psychosomatic Medicine. Karter, Basel, pp. 16–34.

Laumann, E.O., Nicolosi, A., Glasser, D.B. *et al.* (2005) for the GSSAB Investigators' Group Sexual problems among women and men aged 40–80 y: prevalence and correlates identified in the Global Study of Sexual Attitudes and Behaviors. *International Journal of Impotence Research*, **17**, 39–57.

Laumann, E.O., Paik, A. & Rosen, R.C. (1999) Sexual dysfunction in the United States: prevalence and predictors. *Journal of the American Medical Association*, **281**, 537–544.

Leiblum, S.R., Koochaki, P.E., Rodenberg, C.A., Barton, I.P. & Rosen, R.C. (2006) Hypoactive sexual desire disorder in postmenopausal women: US results from the Women's International Study of Health and SExuality (WISHeS). *Menopause*, **13**, 46–56.

Lloyd, E.A. (2005) *The Case of the Female Orgasm: Bias in the Science of Evolution*. Harvard University Press, Cambridge, MA.

Masters, W. & Johnson, V. (1970) *Human Sexual Inadequacy*. Little, Brown, Boston, MA.

McCall, K. & Meston, C. (2006) Cues resulting in desire for sexual activity in women. *Journal of Sexual Medicine*, **3**, 838–852.

Mercer, C.H., Fenton, K.A., Johnson, A.M. *et al.* (2003) Sexual function problems and help seeking behaviour in Britain: national probability sample survey. *British Medical Journal*, **327**, 426–427.

Mitchell, K.R., Mercer, C.H., Wellings, K. & Johnson, A.M. (2009) Prevalence of low sexual desire among women in Britain: associated factors. *Journal of Sexual Medicine*, **6**, 2434–2444.

Oberg, K., Fugl-Meyer, A.R. & Fugl-Meyer, K.S. (2004) On categorization and quantification of women's sexual dysfunctions: an epidemiological approach. *International Journal of Impotence Research*, **16**, 261–269.

Shifren, J.L., Monz, B.U., Russo, P.A., Segreti, A. & Johannes, C.B. (2008) Sexual problems and distress in United States women: prevalence and correlates. *Obstetrics and Gynecology*, **112**, 970–978.

Witting, K., Santtila, P., Varjonen, M. *et al.* (2008) Female sexual dysfunction, sexual distress, and compatibility with partner. *Journal of Sexual Medicine*, **5**, 2587–2599.

CHAPTER 16

Erectile Dysfunction

Geoffrey Hackett

Good Hope Hospital, Birmingham, UK

OVERVIEW

- Diagnosis and management of the underlying causes of ED is at least as important as treating the symptom.
- In around 70% of cases, there will be an endocrine or cardiovascular component to be addressed.
- ED usually occurs 3–5 years before significant cardiovascular events and provides a marker for early intervention and prevention.

Introduction

Erectile dysfunction (ED) has been defined as the persistent inability to attain and/or maintain an erection sufficient for sexual performance. Although ED is not perceived as a life-threatening condition, it is closely associated with many important physical conditions and may affect psychosocial health. As such, ED has a significant impact on the quality of life of patients and their partners.

In the Massachusetts Male Aging Study (MMAS), the prevalence of ED was 52% in non-institutionalized 40- to 70-year-old men in the Boston area: 17.2%, 25.2% and 9.6% for minimal, moderate and complete ED. Prevalence rates are 75% in men with type 2 diabetes. The third National Survey of Sexual Attitudes and Lifestyle survey (Natsal-3) studied 4913 UK men and reported ED rates of 13.4% (45–54), 23.5% (55–64) and 30% (65–74) with only one in four having sought medical help.

Penile erection is a complex neurovascular phenomenon under hormonal control that includes arterial dilatation, trabecular smooth muscle relaxation and activation of the corporeal veno-occlusive mechanism. The risk factors for ED (sedentary lifestyle, obesity, smoking, hypercholesterolaemia and the metabolic syndrome) are very similar to the risk factors for cardiovascular disease.

Initial assessment

Sexual history

A detailed description of the problem, including the duration of symptoms and original precipitants, should be obtained, including:

Predisposing, precipitating and maintaining factors
Treatment interventions along with the response achieved
Quality of morning awakening erections, and spontaneous, masturbatory or partner-related erections
Sexual desire, ejaculatory and orgasmic dysfunction
Previous erectile capacity
Issues around any sexual aversion or sexual pain
Partner issues, for example menopause, low desire or vaginal pain

Physical examinations

All patients should have a focused physical examination. A genital examination is recommended, and this is essential if there is a history of rapid onset of pain, deviation of the penis during tumescence, the symptoms of hypogonadism or other urological symptoms.

The use of validated questionnaires, particularly the International Index of Erectile Function (IIEF) or Sexual Health Inventory for Men (SHIM) may be helpful to assess sexual function domains especially for the impact of treatments and interventions.

Laboratory testing

ED is an independent marker for cardiovascular risk and can be the presenting feature of diabetes, so serum lipids, fasting plasma glucose or ideally HbA1c or IFCC (in light of the recent change in International Diabetes Federation (IDF) criteria) should be measured *in all patients*.

Hypogonadism is a treatable cause of ED that may also make men less responsive, or even non-responsive, to phosphodiesterase type 5 (PDE5) inhibitors, therefore *all men with ED should have serum testosterone measured on a blood sample taken in the morning before 11 a.m.*

Lowed urinary tract symptoms (LUTSs) and benign prostatic hypertrophy (BPH) are closely associated with ED, sharing pathological mechanisms and risk factors. Serum prostate-specific antigen (PSA) should be considered if clinically indicated especially before and during testosterone therapy. Please also see Chapter 10.

ABC of Sexual Health, Third Edition. Edited by Kevan Wylie.
© 2015 John Wiley & Sons, Ltd. Published 2015 by John Wiley & Sons, Ltd.

Cardiovascular disease and ED

Coronary heart disease (CHD) is associated with many of the same risk factors as ED. As the penile arteries are significantly smaller than the main coronary arteries, ED frequently pre-dates coronary artery disease by 3–5 years and early diagnosis is considered a 'window of opportunity' to detect and prevent future cardiac events, especially in *younger men*.

Specialized investigations

Most patients do not need further investigations unless specifically indicated. However, some patients wish to know the cause of their ED. Other indications for specialist investigations include:

- Young patients who have always had difficulty in obtaining and/or sustaining an erection.
- Patients with a history of trauma, including bicycle riding.
- Where an abnormality of the testes or penis is found on examination.
- Patients unresponsive to medical therapies that may desire surgical treatment.

Nocturnal penile tumescence and rigidity (NPTR)

Nocturnal and early awakening erections are a normal physiological event in all men and are associated with the REM pattern of sleep. Nocturnal penile tumescence and rigidity (NPTR) may require hospital admission (especially in forensic cases).

Intracavernous injection test

This outpatient test involves the injection of prostaglandin E1 into the corpora cavernosum of the penis and to assess penile rigidity after 10 min. Its use as a diagnostic test for ED is limited as a positive result can be found in patients with both normal and mild vascular disease. The main use of this test is in the assessment of penile deformities such as Peyronie's disease.

Duplex ultrasound of penile arteries

This radiological investigation which measures blood flow will give an excellent assessment of the penile vasculature in response to an injection of a vasoactive agent but frequently does not influence clinical management.

Arteriography and dynamic infusion cavernosometry or cavernosography

These are highly specialized investigations that are only performed in specific circumstances usually to diagnose primary venous pathology in young men.

Treatment objectives

The primary goal of management of ED is to enable the individual or couple to enjoy a satisfactory sexual experience. This involves:

- Identifying and treating any curable causes of ED.
- Initiating lifestyle change and risk factor modification.
- Providing education and counselling to patients and their partners.

Lifestyle management

Investigations for ED should be aimed at identifying reversible risk factors. Modifications in lifestyle can reduce the risk of ED. Pharmacotherapy should not be withheld on the basis that lifestyle changes have not been made.

Drug-induced ED

A wide range of drugs has been implicated in ED. In many cases, the evidence for drugs having a direct causal relationship with some form of sexual dysfunction is relatively poor.

Cardiovascular drugs and ED

In patients with hypertension and CHD, their ED is usually caused by the medical condition. Patients frequently blame the medication, particularly if there seems to be a temporal relationship. Stopping the offending drug is rarely effective, unless an early therapy switch is made when a definite relationship is found. Thiazides and non-selective beta-blockers have been shown in a number of studies to be associated with ED. Angiotensin receptor blockers (ARBs and not Angiotensin Converting Enzyme Inhibitor (ACEIs) have been shown to have a beneficial effect on ED.

Psychosexual counselling and therapy

Psychosexual therapy either alone or alongside couple's relationship therapy is indicated particularly where the patient and or partner identify significant psychological contribution to the problem or as perpetuating the problem.

Hormonal causes of ED

Endocrine disorders may have a significant effect on sexual function. Their resolution might also lead to the resolution of co-existing sexual dysfunction. Hypogonadism, hyperthyroidism and hyperprolactinaemia are examples of relevant disorders.

Far from being a normal consequence of ageing, hypogonadism is closely associated with obesity and metabolic syndrome. Around 20% of men presenting with ED, and 40% of men with type 2 diabetes will have a total testosterone (TT) of less than 11 nmol/l and be candidates for testosterone replacement therapy (TRT). As a general rule, men with low testosterone as the solitary abnormality are likely to see restoration of sexual desire and erections with TRT, whereas those with other co-morbidities are likely to require specific ED medication in addition. Several recent studies have demonstrated improvement in insulin resistance, visceral fat and metabolic parameters associated with TRT. This is no evidence for increased risk of prostate cancer or BPH.

Oral pharmacotherapy

Drugs that inhibit PDE5 increase arterial blood flow, which leads to smooth muscle relaxation, vasodilation and penile erection. Four potent selective PDE5i inhibitors have been approved to

Table 16.1 PDE5 Inhibitors currently available for treating ED

Treatment	Available in the UK	Formulation and dose available	Food restrictions	How long before sex is tablet taken?	How long is it effective for	Most common side effects
Spedra (avanafil)	2014	Tablet 50,100, 200 mg	No food restriction	30 mins	up to 6 hours	Headache, Flushing, Nasal congestion
Cialis (tadalafil)	2003	Tablet 2.5 mg OAD, 5 mg OAD, 10 and 20 mg	Can be taken with or without food	At least 30 min	Up to 36 h	Headache and dyspepsia
Levitra (vardenafil)	2003	Tablet 5, 10 and 20 mg	Can be taken with or without food, however if taken with high fat meal it may take longer to work	Approxiamtely 25–60 min	Up to 4–5 h	Headache and flushing
Viagra (sildenafil)	1998	Tablet 25, 50 and 100 mg	May take longer to work if taken with food	Approximately 1 h	Up to 4–5 h	Headache and flushing

treat ED – sildenafil, tadalafil, vardenafil and avanafil (Table 16.1). Sildenafil came off patent in 2013 and is considerably less expensive. Changes in NHS regulations in 2014 made generic Sildenafil available at NHS expense to all men with ED. The major difference in these drugs is that sildenafil and vardenafil are relatively short-acting drugs, having a half-life of approximately 4 h, whereas tadalafil has a significantly longer half-life of 17.5 h. PDE5 inhibitors require sexual stimulation in order to facilitate an erection. Tadalafil is licensed for daily use at 2.5 and 5 mg in men where frequent and more spontaneous sex is a priority. At 5 mg daily, it is licensed to treat LUTS/BPH, with the added benefit of improving both conditions, whereas alpha-blockers often impair ejaculatory function, especially if the patient is asked.

Published studies on all four PDE5i inhibitors suggest that 75% of sexual attempts result in successful intercourse with lower efficacy rates in diabetes (50–55%) and after nerve-sparing radical prostatectomy (37–41%). Organic nitrates including nicorandil are absolute contraindications with PDE5i inhibitors due to unpredictable falls in the blood pressure and, potentially, catastrophic hypotension.

Non-responders to PDE5 inhibitors

Approximately 25% of patients do not respond to PDE5 inhibitors. Patients should be exposed to a minimum of 4 (preferably 8) of the highest tolerated dose of at least two drugs with adequate sexual stimulation. Several measures are described to salvage patients, defined as non-responders;

- Re-counselling on proper use, especially the need for direct genital stimulation.
- Optimal treatment of concurrent diseases and re-evaluation for new risk factors.
- Treatment of concurrent hypogonadism. Testosterone regulates the responsiveness of PDE5 inhibitors in the corpus cavernosum and several studies have shown that patients can be salvaged by treating low or low–normal levels.
- Occasionally patients may respond to one drug when another has failed.
- More frequent or daily dosing.
- L-Arginine 2–3 g daily – a nitric oxide precursor shown to be effective, especially combined with PDE5 inhibitors.
- Folic acid 5 mg daily was shown in a single study to enhance the effect of PDE5 inhibitors.

Vacuum erection devices

The principle of vacuum erection devices is simple (Figure 16.1). A cylinder is placed over the penis, air is pumped out with an attached pump and the resulting tumescence is maintained by a constriction ring around the base of the penis.

- Vacuum devices are highly effective in inducing erections regardless of the aetiology of the ED.
- Reported satisfaction rates vary considerably from 35% to 84%
- Long-term usage of vacuum devices is considerably higher than for self-injection therapy.
- Most men who are satisfied with vacuum devices continue to use them long term.
- Adverse effects include bruising, local pain and failure to ejaculate. Partners sometimes report the penis feels cold.
- Serious adverse events are very rare but skin necrosis has been reported.

Vacuum devices are contraindicated in men with bleeding disorders or those taking anticoagulant therapy. They work best if the man and his partner have a positive attitude to them and sufficient time has been spent demonstrating their use. They represent a cost-effective way of treating ED, even though initial costs are high.

Second-line treatment

Intracavernous injection therapy

Intracavernous injection therapy (Figure 16.2) is the most effective form of pharmacotherapy for ED and has been used for more than 20 years. Providing the blood supply is good, an excellent result can be achieved in most men. It does not require an intact nerve supply and can therefore be highly effective after spinal cord injuries and after major pelvic surgery such as after radical prostatectomy. Compliance may be a particular problem if the procedure is not explained clearly and fully at first consultation and if adequate support and follow-up visits are not provided.

Alprostadil

Alprostadil can be used in doses from 5 to 40 μg. The erection occurs typically 5–15 min after penile injection and frequently last 30–40 min. Two or three visits are usually required to ascertain the correct dosage and teach the technique. In patients with limited manual dexterity, the partner may be taught the technique.

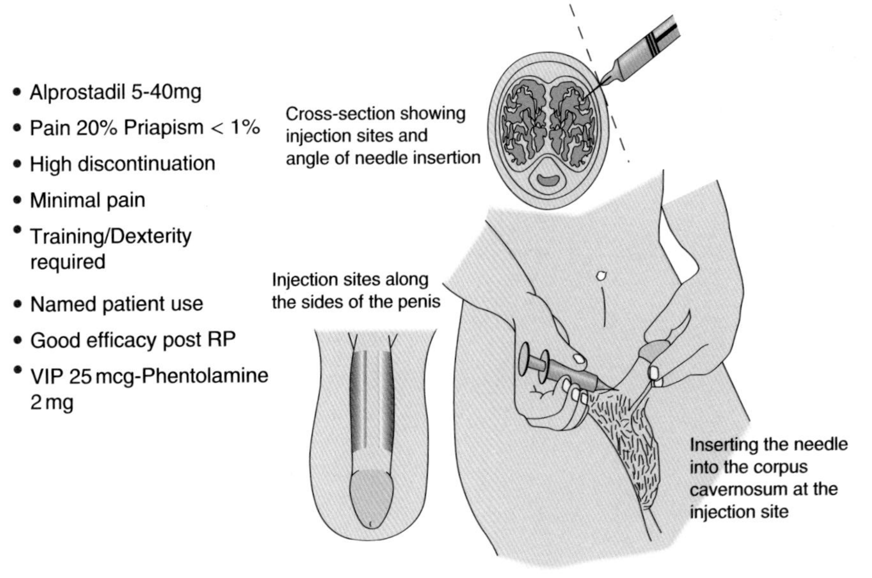

- Alprostadil 5-40mg
- Pain 20% Priapism < 1%
- High discontinuation
- Minimal pain
- Training/Dexterity required
- Named patient use
- Good efficacy post RP
- VIP 25 mcg-Phentolamine 2 mg

Cross-section showing injection sites and angle of needle insertion

Injection sites along the sides of the penis

Inserting the needle into the corpus cavernosum at the injection site

Figure 16.1 Vacuum erection devices

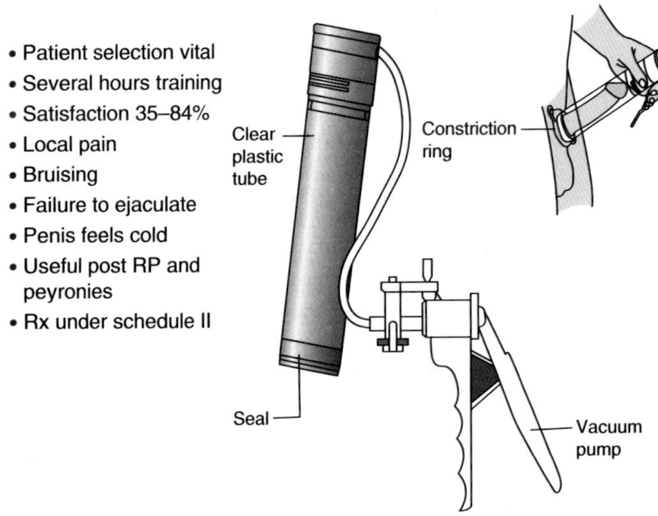

- Patient selection vital
- Several hours training
- Satisfaction 35–84%
- Local pain
- Bruising
- Failure to ejaculate
- Penis feels cold
- Useful post RP and peyronies
- Rx under schedule II

Clear plastic tube

Constriction ring

Seal

Vacuum pump

Figure 16.2 Intra-cavernosal Injection

VIP 25mcg/Phentolamine 2mg mixture

VIP 25mcg/ Phentolamine 2mg mixture is licensed in Scandinavia and expected to be available in 2015 in the UK as Invicorp 2. The potential advantages of the product are reduced levels of pain and greater response to direct stimulation.

Intraurethral alprostadil

A formulation of alprostadil in a medicated pellet is approved for the treatment of ED (Figure 16.3). Patients are told to void to make sure the urethra is moist and then the pellet is inserted into the urethra via a small applicator and then the penis massaged. Medicated urethral system for erection (MUSE) results in erections in approximately 30–60% of patients but continuation rates are disappointing. In clinical practice, only the higher dosages of 500 and 1000 μg are effective.

- Application of a constriction ring at the base of the penis may help in some patients,

- Side-effects include penile pain (30–40%) and dizziness (2–10%).
- Penile fibrosis and priapism are rare (<1%).

A cream formulation of 300mcg of alprostadil (Vitaros), applied to the glans and urethra, became available in 2014.

External low energy shock wave therapy claims to produce neo-vacularization within the corpora and this is available in a few UK centres. Although expensive and labour-intensive, this will be seen as acceptable to many patients seeking a 'cure' for ED. Longer-term studies are required.

Third-line treatment

Penile prosthesis

Penile prostheses should be offered to all patients who are unwilling to consider, failing to respond to or unable to continue with medical therapy or external devices.

Penile prostheses are particularly suitable for those with severe organic ED, especially if the cause is Peyronie's disease or post

- Alprostadil 125–1000 mg
- Good erection of glans
- Needs stimulation
- Modest efficacy
- Pain and irritation
- High discontinuation

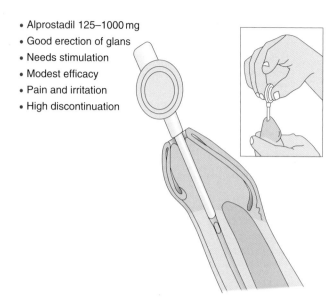

Figure 16.3 Medicated urethral system for erection (MUSE)

priapism. All patients should be given a choice of either a malleable or inflatable prosthesis.

Satisfaction rates of 89% were shown in one series of 434 implants. High rates are mainly due to the improved mechanical reliability of the new devices. Five-year survival of these devices is 93% but a revision rate of 7% per year can be expected.

Peyronie's disease

Peyronie's disease (PD) involves fibrotic plaques with or without curvature, associated with micro-trauma and stress of the tunica albuginea. Prevalence rates are 3–5%, increasing with age. If erections are satisfactory or a successful response with penetration can be achieved with treatment, then surgical treatment is best avoided. Multiple medical treatments have been tried, including vitamin E, potaba, verapamil injections, tamoxifen, oxypentifylline and lithotripsy have shown minimal efficacy and are not recommended by ISSM guidelines. Only Collagenase Clostridium Histolicum (Xiaflex) injections have clinical evidence of efficacy but this is currently an expensive option. Vacuum erection devices (VEDS) can be helpful to improve erections, correct deformity and prevent shortening. If surgical correction is required then a tunical plication (Nesbit procedure) is the treatment of choice for deformities of 60' or less. For greater deformities then plaque excision with grafting is required. If ED cannot be successfully treated prior to surgery, then a penile implant is usually required.

Conclusion

There is now overwhelming evidence that ED is strongly associated with cardiovascular disease, such that newly presenting patients should be thoroughly evaluated for cardiovascular and endocrine risk factors, which should be managed accordingly. Patients attending their primary care physician with chronic cardiovascular disease should be asked about erectile problems. There can no longer be an excuse for avoiding discussions about sexual activity due to embarrassment.

Further reading

Bhasin, S., Cunningham, G.R., Hayes, F.J. *et al.* (2010) Testosterone therapy in men with androgen deficiency syndromes: an Endocrine Society clinical practice guideline. *Journal of Clinical Endocrinology and Metabolism*, **95** (**6**), 2536–2559.

Esposito, K., Giugliano, F., Di Palo, C. *et al.* (2004) Effect of lifestyle changes on erectile dysfunction in obese men: a randomized controlled trial. *JAMA*, **291**, 2978–2984.

Feldman, H.A., Goldstein, I., Hatzichristou, D.G., Krane, R.J. & McKinlay, J.B. (1994) Impotence and its medical and psychosocial correlates: results of the Massachusetts Male Aging Study. *Journal of Urology*, **151**, 54–61.

Hackett, G., Cole, N., Bhartia, M., Kennedy, D., Raju, J. & Wilkinson, P. (2013) Testosterone replacement therapy with long-acting Testosterone Undecanoate improves sexual function and quality-of-life parameters vs. placebo in a population of men with type 2 diabetes. *Journal of Sexual Medicine*, **10** (**6**), 1512–1527.

Hackett, G., Kell, P., Ralph, D. *et al.* (2008) British society for sexual medicine guidelines on the management of erectile dysfunction. *Journal of Sexual Medicine*, **5** (**8**), 1841–1846.

Mitchell, K.R., Mercer, C.H., Ploubidis, G.B. *et al.* (2013) Sexual Function in Britain: findings from the third national survey of Sexual Attitudes and Lifestyles (Natsal-3). *Lancet*, **382** (**9907**), 1830–1844.

Shabsigh, R., Kaufman, J.M., Steidle, C. & Padma-Nathan, H. (2004) Randomized study of testosterone gel as adjunctive therapy to sildenafil in hypogonadal men with erectile dysfunction who do not respond to sildenafil alone. *Journal of Urology*, **172**, 658–663.

CHAPTER 17

Problems of Ejaculation and Orgasm in the Male

Marcel D. Waldinger

Utrecht Institute for Pharmaceutical Sciences, Utrecht University, Utrecht, The Netherlands

> **OVERVIEW**
> - There are four types of premature ejaculation, each with its own characteristics and treatment
> - Drug treatment is particularly indicated for Lifelong and Acquired Premature Ejaculation
> - Acquired delayed ejaculation induced my medication is often reversible after dosage reduction
> - Post Orgasmic Illness Syndrome (POIS) is caused by an auto-immune reaction to the autologous semen of the patient but effective treatment is not yet available.
> - Diagnosis of an ejaculatory disorder combined with explanation of it to the patient is essential for the male's coping with the disorder

Introduction

Ejaculation and orgasm usually occur simultaneously even though ejaculation and orgasm are two separate phenomena. Ejaculation occurs in the genital organs, whereas orgasmic sensation – although related to the genitals – is mainly a cerebral event and involves the whole body. Ejaculation and orgasm problems may cause distress for the man himself and/or his sexual partner. Although in the last two decades, more research has been performed, and particularly premature ejaculation (PE) can effectively be treated, there is still a lack of effective treatment for some ejaculatory disorders. Nevertheless, it is important that ejaculatory and orgasm problems are recognized by the general physician. Informing the patient about the correct diagnosis of his complaints, even when an effective treatment is not (yet) available, may reassure the patient that his complaints are real. Normalizing a reduction of ejaculatory force and volume with advancing age can be very reassuring to a man.

Premature ejaculation

About 20–25% of men are not satisfied with their ejaculation. They perceive it as coming too early. Most of these men do not seek medical help. However, when the ejaculation time is a matter of seconds or just a minute the person feels that he should seek help, but often feels too embarrassed to talk about it with his GP. Therefore, a GP may hardly see a patient complaining of PE. But the reality is different.

There are four types of PE: lifelong PE, acquired PE, subjective PE, and variable PE. Diagnosis of the PE type is essential for a good treatment (Figure 17.1 and Box 17.1).

Lifelong premature ejaculation

In lifelong PE, early ejaculation exists from the first (or nearly first) sexual experiences, usually starting in puberty or adolescence. It occurs with every (or nearly every) female partner in more than 80–90% of events of intercourse. In addition, there is little change in the very short duration of the intravaginal ejaculation latency time (IELT) as men age, or it aggravates in about 30% of the patients at around the age of 30–35 years. Ejaculation occurs within 30–60 s after vaginal penetration with nearly every coitus in more than 90% of men with lifelong PE, whereas about 10–20% of men complaining of lifelong PE ejaculate within 1–2 min. Lifelong PE leads to irritability, annoyance, embarrassment, a decreased feeling of masculinity and sometimes depression. Although the very short IELTs are the major complaint, a lot of men with lifelong PE also complain of easily triggered (early) erections and immediate complete detumescence of the penis after ejaculation. Lifelong PE affects both heterosexual as homosexual men, but hardly any clinical research has been conducted in homosexual men. There are indications that lifelong PE is a neurobiologically and genetically induced ejaculatory disorder. Treatment consists of oral medication and/or topical anaesthetics, often required for a very long time, but always combined with psycho-education and counselling in case of psychological and/or relationship problems. The prevalence of lifelong PE is about 2–3% in the general male population.

Acquired premature ejaculation

In acquired PE, men experience early ejaculations at some point in their life having previously had normal ejaculation experiences. The onset may be either sudden or gradual. The IELT is usually between 1 and 3 min. It may be due to sexual performance anxiety, psychological or relationship problems, but also by prostatitis, hyperthyroidism or erectile difficulties. Acquired PE is the result of a medical and/or psychological disorder and may be cured by medical and/or

ABC of Sexual Health, Third Edition. Edited by Kevan Wylie.

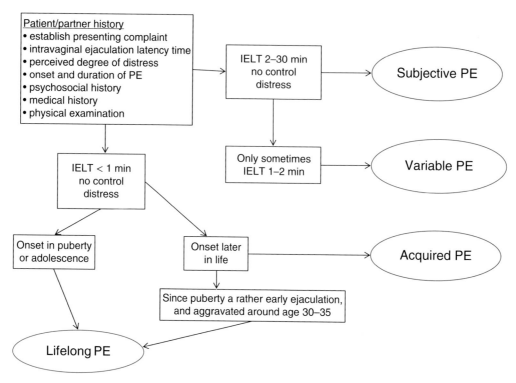

Figure 17.1 An approach to diagnose the four premature ejaculation subtypes

Box 17.1 **Questions to establish the PE subtype**

1 When did you first experience PE?
2 Have you experienced early ejaculation since your first sexual encounters?
3 Did you experience it with most of your sexual partners?
4 What is the time between penetration and ejaculation?
5 How often do you have an early ejaculation with your current partner?
6 Do you feel bothered, annoyed and/or frustrated by your early ejaculation?
7 Is your erection hard enough to penetrate?
8 Do you ever rush intercourse to prevent loss of erection?
9 What is your partner opinion or attitude towards your complaint?

psychological treatment of the underlying disorder, including temporarily oral medication and/or topical anaesthetics. The prevalence of acquired PE is about 4–5% in the general male population.

Subjective premature ejaculation

Men with subjective PE experience or complain of early ejaculation while their ejaculation time, the IELT, is in the normal range of around 2–6 min and sometimes even between 5 and 25 min. Thus, although these men have a normal or even long IELT duration, they still perceive themselves as having PE. As the duration of the IELT in these men is normal, the experience of PE is not related to a medical or neurobiological disturbance. Rather, there is either a misperception of the actual IELT, for various psychological reasons, or the IELT is too short for the female partner to attain an orgasm. Treatment consists of various sorts of psychotherapy and/or topical use of anaesthetics. The prevalence of subjective PE is 5–7% in the general male population.

Variable premature ejaculation

Men with variable PE experience short IELTs only sometimes and only in certain situations. Variable PE is not regarded as a symptom of underlying psychopathology but of normal variation in sexual performance. Treatment of variable PE consists of reassurance and education that this pattern of ejaculatory response is normal and does not require drug treatment or psychotherapy. The prevalence of variable PE is 8–11% in the general male population.

Drug treatment of premature ejaculation

Following assessment (see Chapter 10), there are three evidence-based drug treatment strategies to delay ejaculation: (i) on-demand oral drug treatment, (ii) daily oral drug treatment and (iii) topical application of anaesthetics (Table 17.1). Drug treatment is preferably combined with psycho-education, counselling and should always include information about potential drug-induced side effects. For on-demand drug treatment, two drugs are available: dapoxetine 30–60 mg (1–3 h before intercourse) and clomipramine 20–30 mg (4–6 h before intercourse). Dapoxetine is the only officially registered drug to treat PE. Daily treatment may be performed by off-label use of selective serotonin reuptake inhibitors (SSRIs), such as paroxetine 20 mg/day, sertraline 50–100 mg/day and citalopram 20 mg/day. For topical anaesthetic treatment, off-label use of lidocaine and prilocaine containing creams or sprays are available.

Table 17.1 Drug treatment of lifelong and acquired premature ejaculation

Treatment	Side effects
On-demand oral treatment	
Dapoxetine 30–60 mg, 1–3 h before intercourse	Nausea, dizziness
Clomipramine 20–30 mg, 4–6 h before intercourse (off-label)	Nausea, dry mouth, blurred vision, constipation
Daily oral treatment (off-label)	
Paroxetine hemihydrate 20 mg	Side-effects on the short term (first 3 weeks): fatigue, yawning, slight nausea, perspiration, loose stools
Sertraline 50–100 mg	Side-effects on the long term: increased weight, sometimes decreased libido or erectile difficulties
Citalopram 20 mg	
Fluoxetine 20 mg	
On-demand Topical anaesthetics (off-label)	
Cream with lidocaine and prilocaine	Erectile difficulties, numbness penis
Spray lidocaine	

Additional information for the patient

Very rarely SSRIs may cause penile anaesthesia or hypoesthesia. The patient should be informed that in case of penile anaesthesia the SSRI should be discontinued

In case the patient want to stop taking an SSRI, this should occur very gradually in 4–6 weeks in order to prevent the occurrence of an SSRI discontinuation syndrome

In case of a wish for pregnancy, it is better to postpone SSRI treatment or to discontinue the use of an SSRI as there are some indications that SSRI treatment of a male may affect spermatozoa

Delayed ejaculation

Lifelong delayed ejaculation

In lifelong delayed ejaculation men complain of an unwanted marked delay or even absence of ejaculation in partnered sexual activity and/or during mastubation, persistently occurring since the first sexual contacts in puberty or adolescence. These men usually report prolonged thrusting to achieve orgasm (often) to the point of exhaustion or genital discomfort of the partner. They usually discontinue intercourse, often to frustration of the man himself and/or his sexual partner. Sometimes, the patient is able to ejaculate by masturbation but only after great efforts. There is no evidence-based treatment for lifelong delayed ejaculation, and there is currently no drug for safe human usage that facilitates ejaculation. Various psychotherapeutic treatments, such as behavioural therapy, have been investigated with varying degrees of success. The prevalence is not well known but is estimated to be about 1% of the general male population.

Acquired delayed ejaculation

In acquired delayed ejaculation, men report difficulties in getting an ejaculation somewhere in life after a period of relatively normal sexual function. Acquired delayed ejaculation may be caused by medication, psychological problems and ageing (Table 17.2). With increasing age, age-related loss of the fast conducting peripheral sensory nerves of the genitals may induce a delayed ejaculation. Between the age of 55 and 85 years, the prevalence of acquired delayed ejaculation increases from 16% to 33%.

Table 17.2 Causes of acquired delayed ejaculation

Psychological
Psychological trauma
Lack of sexual stimulation (i.e. inadequate technique, lack of attention to sexual stimuli)

Somatic
Androgen deficiency
Spinal injury
Lumbar sympathectomy
Abdomino perineal surgery
Multiple sclerosis
Diabetic neuropathy

Medication
Selective serotonin reuptake inhibitors (SSRIs)
Tricyclic antidepressants
Antipsychotics
α-sympathicolytics
Treatment of acquired PE consists of treatment of underlying cause and in case of medication reducing the dosage or discontinuation of the drug and switching to an antidepressant with less ejaculation delaying effects (bupropion XR, mirtazapine, agomelatine, or vortioxetine)

Post-orgasmic illness syndrome

Men with Post-orgasmic illness syndrome (POIS) become ill within a few minutes to a few hours after ejaculation. Their complaints consist of getting a flu-like feeling, extreme fatigue or exhaustion, weakness of musculature, feverishness, perspiration, mood disturbances and/or irritability, memory difficulties, concentration problems, incoherent speech, congestion of nose and/or itching eyes. The number of complaints varies and not all these symptoms together are required for the diagnosis of POIS. However, for the diagnosis it is required that the symptoms occur after each ejaculation that is initiated by coitus, masturbation, or spontaneous during sleep. The complaints of a POIS 'attack' last for about 2–7 days and disappear spontaneously. In primary POIS, the POIS attacks are present since the first ejaculations in puberty. In secondary POIS, the POIS attacks start later in life. Men affected by POIS tend to avoid these symptoms as much as possible. They either abstain from sexual activities or schedule sexual activities to episodes without important social or work obligations. POIS leads to often severe psychosocial difficulties, relationship problems, divorce, depressive feelings and sometimes suicidal thoughts. This may become aggravated by non-understanding of partners, colleagues and medical specialists, as POIS is still an unknown disorder in general medicine. There are strong indications that POIS is caused by a systemic autoimmune reaction to the male's own semen as soon this is triggered by ejaculation. This autoimmune reaction produces certain cytokines that trigger the symptoms of POIS. Although 3–5 years regular desensitization with very diluted auto-semen is a treatment option, there is currently no evidence-based treatment to cure POIS. The prevalence of POIS is unknown, but it is probably not such a rare disorder.

Restless genital syndrome in the male

Men with restless genital syndrome (ReGS) complain of a persistent urge or sensation in the genital area to ejaculate in absence of an erection or sexual desire. This urge is experienced as unwanted and is accompanied by irritating genital feelings that are difficult to translate in words. It may be accompanied by complaints of an overactive bladder and/or restless legs. Although ReGS in the male has hardly been investigated, it is presumably caused by a neuropathy of the dorsal nerve of the penis, which is an endbranch of the pudendal nerve. Currently, there is no evidence-based treatment for ReGS in the male. However, clonazepam 0.5 mg/day and/or pelvis muscle exercises are treatment options to explore. The prevalence of ReGS in the male is unknown, but presumably very low.

Anhedonic ejaculation

Men with anhedonic ejaculation report to have lost the feeling or sensation of an orgasm during ejaculation. There is a real paucity of literature on this phenomenon. Although it has always been attributed to psychological problems, medical underlying pathology (urethritis, prostatitis, α-blockers, antidepressants, pelvic tumour, neuropathy) should be excluded. The prevalence of anhedonic ejaculation is unknown.

Retrograde ejaculation

Men with retrograde ejaculation ejaculate with preserved orgasm but without semen production. In retrograde ejaculation, semen passes into the bladder during ejaculation due either to internal bladder sphincter incompetence or discoordination between the bladder neck closure and the external sphincter relaxation. It may be caused by α-blockers used for the treatment of lower urinary tract symptoms (LUTS) or benign prostatic hypertrophy (BPH), or invasive BPH procedures such as transurethral resection of prostate (TURP) or laser coagulations. Diabetic neuropathy, spinal cord injury and extended retroperitoneal lymphadenectomy (RLA) have also been related to retrograde ejaculation. For the diagnosis, the presence of sperm in post-orgasmic urine should be confirmed.

Painful ejaculation

Pain or a burning sensation during ejaculation is called painful ejaculation or odynorgasmia. The pain, which can be very severe and frightening, can be felt between the anus and the genitals, in the testes, or in the urethra and may lead to the avoidance of sex. Painful ejaculation may have a number of causes, such as inflammation (seminal vesiculitis, acute prostatitis, chronic prostatitis/chronic pelvic pain syndrome, urethritis), sexually-transmitted infections, benign prostatic hypertrophy, nerve damage in the penis, chronic pain in the pelvis, obstruction in the ejaculatory duct system, prostatectomy, pelvic radiation, prostate cancer, and very rarely certain antidepressants. The cause of painful ejaculation may also remain unknown.

Treatment of painful ejaculation depends on the cause, which is established by a thorough medical examination, and if required analysis of a sample of urine or semen. In case of an inflammation medication should be prescribed. In case of a sexually-transmitted infection antibiotics are required and in case of an antidepressant changing the medication should be considered.

Low ejaculate volume

The normal volume of the semen or ejaculate fluid is between 3–5 ml. The ejaculate volume consists of seminal fluid and spermatozoa. The amount is dependent of the activity of the prostate gland, seminal vesicles and testicles. But it varies also with frequency of sexual activity, physical condition and mood. Only around 1% of the volume consists of sperm cells.

Low ejaculate volume is called hypospermia. It may be due to infections, hypogonadism, retrograde ejaculation, obstruction in a seminal vesicle or ejaculatory duct, varicose vein (varicocele), failure of emission by nerve damage, seminal vesicle cyst, congenital bilateral absence of the vas deferens CBAVD, or hypoplasia of the seminal vesicles. However, it may also be due to a short abstinence period of the male or incomplete collection. Collection of the semen should be performed after 2–3 days of abstinence. A careful history and physical examination, combined with some basic investigations may be helpful in identifying the underlying cause, although none of the semen analysis findings are specific for the causes of low ejaculate volume. Nevertheless, normal semen parameters may be found in partial retrograde ejaculation. Low fructose in semen may indicate problems in the prostatic pathways or ejaculatory duct obstruction. And low semen pH may indicate problems of the seminal vesicles.

Further reading

Althof, S.E., Abdo, C.H.N., Dean, J. et al. (2010) International Society for Sexual Medicine's guidelines for the diagnosis and treatment of premature ejaculation. *Journal of Sexual Medicine*, 7, 2947–2969.

Roberts, M. & Jarvi, K. (2009) Steps in the investigation and management of low semen volume in the infertile man. *Canadian Urological Association Journal*, 3, 479–485.

Serefoglu, E.C., Yaman, O., Cayan, S. et al. (2011) Prevalence of the complaint of ejaculating prematurely and the four premature ejaculation syndromes: results from the Turkish Society of Andrology Sexual Health Survey. *Journal of Sexual Medicine*, **8** (**2**), 540–548.

Waldinger, M.D. (2007) Premature ejaculation: definition and drug treatment. *Drugs*, **67**, 547–568.

Waldinger, M.D. (2013) Ejaculatio praecox, erectio praecox, and detumescentia praecox as symptoms of a hypertonic state in lifelong premature ejaculation: a new hypothesis. *Pharmacology Biochemistry and Behavior*, **121**, 88–101., [Epub ahead of print]

Waldinger, M.D., Meinardi, M.M. & Schweitzer, D.H. (2011) Hyposensitization therapy with autologous semen in two Dutch caucasian males: beneficial effects in Postorgasmic Illness Syndrome (POIS; Part 2). *Journal of Sexual Medicine*, **8**, 1171–1176.

Waldinger, M.D., Venema, P.L., van Gils, A.P., de Lint, G.J. & Schweitzer, D.H. (2011) Stronger evidence for small fiber sensory neuropathy in restless genital syndrome: two case reports in males. *Journal of Sexual Medicine*, **8**, 325–330.

Waldinger, M.D., Zwinderman, A.H., Schweitzer, D.H. & Olivier, B. (2004) Relevance of methodological design for the interpretation of efficacy of drug treatment of premature ejaculation: a systematic review and meta-analysis. *International Journal of Impotence Research*, **16**, 369–381.

CHAPTER 18

Problems of Orgasm in the Female

Sharon J. Parish

Weill Cornell Medical Collage, New York, USA
New York Presbyterian Hospital/Westchester Division, New York, USA

OVERVIEW

- Female orgasm disorder (FOD) occurs in 5–10% of women
- FOD is characterized by persistent or recurrent difficulty, delay in or absence of orgasm in nearly all sexual encounters, which causes personal distress, for 6 months or more
- Clinical evaluation includes assessment of the patient's self-reported orgasm difficulties and a biopsychosocial assessment of common factors associated with FOD
- Biological treatment options include addressing underlying medical conditions and managing medication-induced FOD by waiting for tolerance, dose reduction, augmentation or switching strategies
- Effective non-pharmacological strategies for addressing psychosocial and cultural causes of FOD include psychological counselling, cognitive behavioural therapy, couples training and mindfulness practices.

Box 18.1 **Definition and classification of FOD**

Marked persistent or recurrent delay in, infrequency of, or absence of orgasm or marked reduced intensity of orgasmic sensations in nearly all (75–100%) sexual encounters for at least 6 months
Lifelong versus acquired types
Generalized versus situational types
Despite lack of high self-reported arousal
Interferes with relationship sexual satisfaction

Introduction and definitions

Orgasm difficulties can affect the patient's well-being, self-esteem and relationship satisfaction. Female orgasm disorder (FOD) is defined in diagnostic and statistical manual (DSM-5) as the marked persistent or recurrent delay in, infrequency of or absence of orgasm or marked reduced intensity of orgasmic sensations. The DSM IV-R articulated that these difficulties in orgasm must occur following a normal sexual excitement phase and cause personal distress. The DSM-5 criteria called for a precise duration and frequency and deleted 'following normal sexual excitement phase'. While it is difficult to reach orgasm without adequate sexual excitement, this omission may present some difficulty for the clinician in differentiating orgasm disorders from excitement problems. According to this more recent definition, the symptoms should have persisted for at least 6 months and occur 'quite often' in nearly all (>75%) of sexual encounters, distinguishing orgasm dysfunction from more episodic or transient difficulties (Box 18.1).

Orgasm disorders have traditionally been divided into lifelong versus acquired problems and generalized versus situational impairments. In the lifelong subtype, the woman has never reached orgasm, whereas the acquired type occurs after a period of normal functioning. In generalized FOD, a women is anorgasmic with all types of stimulation, situations or partners, whereas the situational subtype FOD occurs in specific circumstances or conditions. In lifelong situational FOD, the woman can only reach orgasm in some circumstances (masturbation or manual clitoral stimulation), but not in others (in the presence of her partner or with intercourse). The DSM-5 scheme requires the clinician to assess whether a woman has ever reached orgasm and whether her level of her distress is mild, moderate or severe.

An international classification committee commission by the American Urological Association Foundation defined FOD as lack of, delay of, or diminished orgasm from any kind of stimulation, *despite the lack of high self-reported arousal*. The International Classification of Diseases (ICDs) 10 specifies that FOD occurs consistently enough to interfere with the woman's ability to participate in a sexual relationship the way she would like.

The diagnosis of FOD is based on the clinician's judgement that the woman's capacity to experience orgasm is less than expected for her age, prior sexual experience and adequacy of sexual stimulation in her sexual encounters.

Prevalence

There are wide estimates of the prevalence of FODs, ranging from 10% to 42%. Approximately 10% of women do not report experience of orgasm. Interpretation of prevalence and incidence

---

ABC of Sexual Health, Third Edition. Edited by Kevan Wylie.
© 2015 John Wiley & Sons, Ltd. Published 2015 by John Wiley & Sons, Ltd.

rates of FOD requires recognition that there is a wide of 'normal' for the acquisition of orgasmic capacity. A women's first orgasmic experience can occur before puberty or well into adulthood. Women's incidence of ever having an orgasm increases with age as they experience a wide variety of sexual stimulation. Also, women are more likely to consistently experience orgasm with masturbation than during partnered sexual activity. The prevalence of primary lifelong orgasm disorders, defined as a woman having never reached orgasm by any means, is approximately 10%. In women with FOD, up to 31% report other sexual difficulties, with arousal and lubrication problems being the most common.

While women report that the ability to reach orgasm is important to overall sexual satisfaction, orgasm and satisfaction may not be linked in every woman or in every sexual experience.

Anatomy and physiology

While some women respond preferentially to clitoral or vaginal stimulation, evidence suggests the clitoral complex is stimulated during vaginal penetration. The internal clitoris, composed of clitoral bodies and bulbs, is 10× or larger than the glans clitoris; together they make up the 'clitoral complex'.

As women age, they normally experience changes in their physiological sexual response. Changes include decreased vaginal muscle tension and expansion of the vaginal vault, delay in reaction time in the clitoris, and lack of breast size increase during stimulation. When oestrogen levels decline with menopause, women may experience atrophic changes and dyspareunia. Although orgasmic capacity is retained with age, there is a decrease in the number and intensity of vaginal contractions; consequently, women may require more intense or direct clitoral stimulation, such as with a vibrator.

Pathophysiology

Once a female learns how to reach orgasm, she will usually not lose that capacity unless problems intervene, such as ineffective sexual communication, a relationship issue, a traumatic experience, a mood disorder or an organic factor.

Biological risk factors

FOD may be the result of insufficient central hormonal sexual excitatory processes (dopamine, oxytocin, melanocortin and noradrenaline) or of increased sexual inhibitory processes (opioid, endocannabinoid and serotonergic systems).

Physiological factors affecting a woman's experience of orgasm include medical conditions, medications and substances of abuse, as well as genetic factors (Box 18.2). Medical problems causing FOD include vascular disease, diabetic neuropathy, multiple sclerosis, genital mutilation or complications from genital surgery, pelvic nerve damage from radical hysterectomy and pelvic trauma. Approximately 50% of spinal cord injured women maintain their orgasmic capacity; preservation depends on the level, completeness and type of lesion. Women with hormonal issues such as thyroid disease, low testosterone or diminished oestrogen resulting in vulvovaginal atrophy are more likely to report orgasmic dysfunction.

Box 18.2 Organic factors that may affect orgasm

Adrenal insufficiency (Addison's disease, adrenalectomy, oophorectomy)
Degenerative arthritis
Diabetes mellitus
Disc disease of lumbosacral spine
Oestrogen deficiency
Female genital mutilation
Hypopituitarism
Hypothyroidism and hyperthyroidism
Hyperlipidaemia
Hypertension
Multiple sclerosis
Neurogenic bladder
Spinal cord lesions
Peripheral neuropathy (alcoholic, diabetic)
Pelvic fracture and radiation
Pelvic or urologic surgery
Vascular disease

Box 18.3 Medications/substance that may affect orgasm

Alcohol (high dose)
Amphetamines
Androgens
Antihistamines
Antihypertensives
Antipsychotics
Cocaine
Opiates
Serotonin reuptake inhibitors
Tobacco
Tricyclic antidepressants

Medical and psychiatric conditions that are co-morbid and correlated with FOD include depression, anxiety, urinary incontinence, fibromyalgia and arthritis, as well as poor overall health status. Excessive alcohol use and opiate misuse are associated with orgasm difficulties.

Medications such as selective serotonin reuptake inhibitors (SSRIs), cardiovascular drugs, mood stabilizers and antihypertensives can cause pharmacologically induced sexual dysfunction (Box 18.3). In women taking SSRIs, at least 37% complain of delayed or absent orgasm.

Psychological and socio-cultural risk factors

Sexual excitation and sexual inhibition imbalance resulting in FOD may be the consequence of psychosocial issues. These include sexual inexperience, body image, ineffective sexual communication, a traumatic relationship experience, fatigue, emotional concerns, past trauma and abuse history, cultural and religious prohibitions and feeling excess pressure to have sex (e.g. infertility). Other common aetiologies resulting in FOD include psychological responses such as spectatoring (obsessive self-observation during sex), unresolved marital conflict, religious guilt, shame and fear of pregnancy. FOD may also be related to male partner sexual dysfunctions, such as erectile dysfunction or premature ejaculation.

Diagnosis

The clinical diagnosis of FOD is established by the clinician's biopsychosocial evaluation. While there are physiological changes during orgasm in the brain, central and systemic hormones, the genito-pelvic region, and pelvic floor muscles, there is substantial variability across all women. Thus, the diagnosis of FOD is based on the history of the women's self-report. The interviewer can discuss the duration, circumstances, and distress and frustration related to orgasm dysfunction, as well as health, cognitive, behavioural, relationship, partner and environmental factors, as discussed above.

In assessing whether a woman has this disorder, the clinician should consider the wide variation in the type or intensity of stimulation that triggers orgasm. Many women require clitoral stimulation to reach orgasm, others require vaginal penetration, and some respond to both forms of stimulation. The clinician should appraise a woman's orgasmic capacity in the context of her age and sexual experience. With situational disorders, the clinician should assess the female's satisfaction and concern for the problem.

Evaluation

Physiological approaches to improving orgasmic function focus on ruling out contributing medical and medication causes. The physical examination may be utilized to assess a woman's overall health status, hormonal issues such as thyroid disease, pelvic floor and vulvovaginal condition.

Blood testing should be considered to assess ovarian, pituitary and thyroid function. Blood tests may include sex hormone levels such as testosterone, sex hormone binding globulin, dihydrotestosterone, luteinising hormone (LH), follicle stimulating hormone (FSH), oestradiol, progesterone, prolactin and thyroid stimulating hormone (TSH).

Treatment

The underlying cause of FOD is often multifactorial, thus treatment should be multifaceted and address those factors amenable to intervention.

In women who have FOD due to hormonal changes associated with menopause, research trials have demonstrated the restoration of sexual responsiveness with testosterone replacement, currently available only for off-label use. While oestrogen and/or progestin trial results regarding improvement in orgasmic function have been mixed, these hormonal treatments have demonstrated efficacy in treating other postmenopausal symptoms.

There are no FDA-approved pharmacological treatments for FOD. Women with FOD related to use of an SSRI may respond to waiting for tolerance to develop, a weekend drug holiday or to a gradual decrease in dose. The latter two strategies may result in a

> **Box 18.4 Psychological and behavioural interventions for FOD**
>
> Psychosocial counselling for relationship issues, stress, religious and cultural conflicts
> Cognitive behavioural therapy to address negative attitudes, shame and guilt
> Management of co-morbid desire and arousal sexual dysfunctions
> Treatment of underlying mood and anxiety disorders
> Referral for intensive therapy for history of trauma or sexual abuse
> Interventions for alcohol and substance misuse
> Directed masturbation training (erotica, vibrators)
> Couples counselling regarding sexual positioning (women on top, coital alignment)
> Training in Kegel exercises and pelvic floor physical therapy
> Guidance with sensate focus exercises
> Recommendation of mindfulness strategies and yoga exercises

recurrence of symptoms (depression, anxiety) or SSRI withdrawal symptoms, and patients must be appropriately counselled and closely monitored. Another strategy is to continue the daily SSRI and add a second agent such as bupropion. Alternatively, the SSRI can be substituted with a dopamine agonist antidepressant such as bupropion. Limited data suggest that the use of sildenafil as an episodic antidote may also be an effective strategy for treatment of emergent SSRI-induced FOD. Small studies show that those who do develop an orgasm disorder following spinal cord injury may respond to sildenafil.

Psychological approaches to FOD focus on encouraging the woman exploring psychosocial factors such as hypoactive sexual desire disorder, depression, poor arousal, anxiety, fatigue, emotional concerns, past abuse, cultural and religious prohibitions, relationship issues or a partner's sexual dysfunction (Box 18.4). Cognitive and behavioural strategies for FOD include directed masturbation training combined with vibrators and fantasy material; Kegel exercises and pelvic floor physical therapy; sensate focus exercises (graded exposure from non-sexual to sexual touching) and sexual positions that allow women control of stimulation and pelvic thrusting.

During sex therapy couples can learn to use manual or vibrator stimulation, the female-above position or coital alignment ('riding high' variation of the missionary position) during intercourse to allow for greater stimulation of the clitoris. Sex therapy for FOD may utilize mindfulness strategies and yoga exercises and also educate the woman to examine and adjust expectations of orgasm.

Further reading

Bancroft, J., Graham, C.A., Janssen, E. & Sanders, S.A. (2009) The dual control model: current status and future directions. *Journal of Sex Research*, **46**, 121–142.

Basson, R., Berman, J., Burnett, A. *et al.* (2000) Report of the international consensus of development conference on female sexual dysfunction: definitions and classifications. *Journal of Urology*, **163**, 888–893.

Basson, R., Leiblum, S., Brotto, L. *et al.* (2003) Definitions of women's sexual dysfunction reconsidered: Advocating expansion and revision. *Journal of Psychosomatic Obstetrics and Gynaecology*, **24**, 221–229.

Clayton, A., Pradko, J.F., Croft, H.A. *et al.* (2002) Prevalence of sexual dysfunction among newer antidepressants. *Journal of Clinical Psychiatry*, **63**, 357–366.

Dunn, K.M., Cherkas, L.F. & Spector, T.D. (2005) Genetic influences on variation in female orgasmic function: a twin study. *Biology Letters*, **1**, 260–263.

Goldstein, I. (2007) Current management strategies of the postmenopausal patient with sexual health problems. *Journal of Sexual Medicine*, **4** (**Suppl 3**), 235–253.

IsHak, W.W., Bokarius, A., Jeffrey, J.K., Davis, M.C. & Bakhta, Y. (2010) Disorders of orgasm in women: a literature review of etiology and current treatments. *Journal of Sexual Medicine*, **7**, 3254–3268.

Laan, E., Rellini, A.H. & Barnes, T. (2013) Standard operating procedures for female orgasmic disorder: consensus of the International Society for Sexual Medicine. *Journal of Sexual Medicine*, **10**, 74–82.

Shifren, J.L., Monz, B.U., Russo, P.A., Segreti, A. & Johannes, C.B. (2008) Sexual problems and distress in United States women: prevalence and correlates. *Obstetrics and Gynecology*, **112** (**5**), 970–978.

Sungur, M.Z. & Gündüz, A. (2014) A comparison of DSM-IV-TR and DSM-5 definitions for sexual dysfunctions: critiques and challenges. *Journal of Sexual Medicine*, **11** (**2**), 364–373.

CHAPTER 19

Sexual Pain Disorders – Male and Female

Melissa A. Farmer[1,2,3], Seth Davis[2] and Yitzchak M. Binik[3]

[1]Feinberg School of Medicine, Northwestern University, Chicago, IL, USA
[2]Faculty of Medicine, University of Toronto, Toronto, ON, Canada
[3]Department of Psychology, McGill University and Sex and Couple Therapy Service, McGill University Health Center, QC, Canada

---

OVERVIEW

- Genito-pelvic pain, which interferes with sexual and non-sexual activities, represents a spectrum of pain conditions
- Genito-pelvic pain impairs sexual functioning by driving negative cognitive/emotional responses and interpersonal conflict
- The multidisciplinary management of genito-pelvic pain is a realistic goal, whereas a focus on 'curing' the pain is unhelpful for physicians and patients
- Unhelpful cognitive/emotional coping strategies require reframing to enhance a patient's ability to adapt to pain
- Comorbid sexual dysfunction can be caused by physiological, psychological and interpersonal factors.

Introduction

The conceptualization of sexual pain has evolved rapidly over the past decade. Pain that was once attributed to sexual neuroses has been accepted as a multifaceted clinical reality that affects between 8 and 15% of women and 5–18% of men. The symptoms that characterize the so-called sexual pain disorders are not restricted to sexual interactions, and this rationale underlies the ongoing efforts to establish these conditions as pain syndromes, rather than variants of sexual dysfunction. Before the release of DSM-5, sexual pain disorders included dyspareunia (pain during sexual intercourse or genital contact in men and women) and vaginismus (fear and avoidance of genital penetration, with possibility of vaginal muscle spasms in women). These disorders have been replaced by genito-pelvic pain/penetration disorder (GPPPD), which captures the clinically significant and frequently comorbid symptoms of genital pain, fear/anxiety (as well as behavioural avoidance) of sexual intercourse, and pelvic floor muscle tension. Importantly, the characterization of GPPPD is expected to simplify the assessment process and provide more straightforward directives regarding treatment strategies (e.g. focusing on psychological factors, pelvic floor muscle function and/or urogynaecological disturbances). This constellation of symptoms is supported by psychological theories

of pain as an experience that perpetuates fear/anxiety of future pain and generates muscle tension near painful regions of the body, thereby reinforcing avoidance of pain-provoking activities, such as sexual intercourse.

Whereas GPPPD can manifest in non-sexual situations (e.g. sitting, walking, bicycle riding, during urination), it can also cause debilitating effects on an individual's sexual life. GPPPD is the only sexual dysfunction that can be 'inflicted' by one's intimate partner, and as a result, genito-pelvic pain can facilitate devastating negative sexual self-appraisals ('I am not a real woman if I cannot have sex without pain'), as well as aversive interpersonal experiences between the sufferer and partner. However, these negative sexual effects are highly dependent on the unique pattern of genito-pelvic pain, an individual's awareness of how the body and mind react to pain, as well as the couple's response to the pain.

Pain history

Considering the heterogeneous nature of pelvic pain, the pain interview is an important tool to establish a clear understanding of the pain being presented (Table 19.1). The pain interview can provide critical information to understand the diagnostic category, potential underlying mechanisms, precipitating and maintaining factors and consequences of pain, thus providing a guideline for multidisciplinary treatment. The pain interview is also a unique opportunity to understand the cognitive and behavioural factors that may maintain or exacerbate pain.

Although many genito-pelvic pain syndromes share underlying features, the European Association of Urology has described potentially distinct pain subtypes based on the affected organ(s). Even when a specific pain syndrome is clinically definable, the clinician should be aware of, and assess, the various different systems that likely contribute to the pain experience (refer to Table 19.2).

When assessing the temporal aspects of pain, it is tempting to try to define a precipitating factor or event that caused the pain. Even if a specific event does exist, the patient may not be able to identify it, and the causal factors that initiated pain may not be the most important ones that continue to maintain the pain.

The character (quality) and location of pain may provide important clues as to the underlying mechanism(s); however, it is important to be aware that pain may radiate from another location. For instance, bladder pain may elicit perineal sensitivity to

---

ABC of Sexual Health, Third Edition. Edited by Kevan Wylie.
© 2015 John Wiley & Sons, Ltd. Published 2015 by John Wiley & Sons, Ltd.

Table 19.1 An approach to the pain history

Temporal questions

1 Time since pain began?
2 At what age did pain begin?
3 Frequency of pain?
4 Pain pattern (cyclic, constant, provoked, spontaneous)?
5 Length of pain symptoms?

Pain character/quality

1 Intensity (0–10 scale)?
2 Pain location?
3 Pain radiation?
4 Pain quality?
5 Other accompanying symptoms?

Pain causes

1 Pain triggers?
2 Provoked or idiopathic?
3 Percentage of pain occurrence with provoking activities?
4 Aggravating/relieving factors?
5 Past surgery or trauma to area?
6 For women, use of hormonal birth control, parity?

Consequences of pain

1 Interference with daily life?
2 Interference with relationship/sexual health?
3 Behavioural response to pain?
4 Medication use?

Psychosocial aspects of pain

1 Sexually active?
2 Sexual dysfunction secondary to pain?
3 Anxiety/catastrophizing/depression about pain?
4 Current or past sexual abuse?

touch and pressure. Triggers of pain, such as movement, urination or vaginal penetration, may also provide useful information. However, for many patients, pain is idiopathic or preceding factors may be difficult to identify. In this case, the pain diary may be of particular use.

Finally, the pain interview is the optimal method for understanding the inter-relationship between pain, psychological factors and sexual functioning. It is essential to assess how the individual interprets pain (e.g. it may elicit fear of further injury or trauma), as well as the behaviours the patient engages in to cope with the pain. If the pain is associated with sex, or if comorbid sexual dysfunction is present, it is important to understand the temporal relationship between sexual activity and pain, both during specific sexual encounters, as well as historically. If the patient is in a relationship, the partner's response to pain, as well as the impact of pain on the dyadic relationship, should be assessed. Finally, a history of sexual abuse should be assessed, although positive findings should be used as part of the psychosocial profile, and not as a causal factor.

Physical examination

The initial goal of the pain assessment should be to evaluate whether there is an ongoing disease process that may better explain the pain

(refer to pain assessment algorithm in Figure 19.1). There is often a fear shared by many patients that pain may indicate a more nefarious underlying disease process, such as cancer. If disease is detected, the first step should be to treat the specific disease process and then reassess whether treatment has resolved the pain. Once disease has been ruled out, it is still advisable to assess whether acute or recurrent trauma, infection and/or inflammation are present. These symptoms may be present in a small number of patients; however, even when these issues are resolved, the pain may continue. Important factors to rule out include infection/inflammation of the prostate in men, bladder inflammation in men and women, and recurrent vaginal or urinary tract infections.

Once acute processes have been ruled out, a holistic approach to patient care is likely to provide the maximum improvement. This approach should adopt a biopsychosocial approach to assessment, as there are often a variety of contributing and maintaining factors underlying pain. The UPOINT(S) phenotyping system – which is an abbreviation for *U*rological, *P*sychological, *O*rgan-specific, *I*nfectious, *N*eurological, *T*enderness of the pelvic floor, and *S*exual systems – is ideal for evaluating male and female GPPPD, as it assesses pain on these diverse psychological and biomedical domains to guide treatment for the affected domains (Table 19.3). The hypothesis underlying the UPOINT(S) system is that, for the vast majority of genito-pelvic pain patients, there can be multiple distinct systems involved in causing and perpetuating the pain. Even if a single system may have been involved initially, as the pain becomes chronic, more systems may become involved in the maintenance of pain. Each domain of the UPOINT(S) system should be addressed separately and can be coded with a yes/no dichotomy. If a patient is found to be positive on a domain, specific treatment designed for that domain should be combined with treatments that are utilized for other co-existing positive domains.

Keeping a pain diary

A pain diary is a useful tool to help characterize an individual's pain, over time. The goal of a pain diary is to monitor and record the circumstances surrounding the pain experience, including events or situations that immediately preceded pain onset, the individual's cognitive appraisal of the pain, and his or her emotional response. By charting daily fluctuations in pain, mood, stress levels and activities, an individual can identify patterns that are associated with pain. Importantly, individuals can typically change aspects of their environment, as well as their cognitive-emotional responses to pain, thereby providing a sense of control over the pain. This exercise, in itself, can be therapeutic.

Sexual dysfunction and the couple

Genito-pelvic pain can potentially disrupt or inhibit all aspects of the sexual response cycle, including blunting of sexual desire/motivation, inhibiting sexual arousal and vaginal lubrication, impairing the capacity to achieve orgasm, provoking pain at and immediately after ejaculation, as well as leaving residual pelvic pain for minutes to hours after sexual activity. As a result, the incidence of comorbid sexual dysfunction, for those

Table 19.2 Potential syndromes underlying genito-pelvic pain in men and women

Affected systems	Pelvic pain syndromes	Symptoms
Urological	Prostate pain syndrome Chronic prostatitis Prostatodynia	Recurrent pain reproduced in prostate, without proven infection or pathology
	Bladder pain syndrome Interstitial cystitis	Recurrent pain in bladder accompanied by worsening on filling, nocturia or urgency/frequency
	Scrotal/testicular/epididymal pain syndrome	Recurring localized pain without signs of infection or trauma
	Penile pain syndrome	Recurrent pain in penis, but not urethra without signs of infection or trauma
	Urethral pain syndrome	Recurrent pain in urethra without signs of infection or trauma. Found in men and women
	Post-vasectomy scrotal pain syndrome	Chronic scrotal pain following vasectomy. As often as 1% following vasectomy
Gynaecological	Vulvar pain syndrome	Vulvar pain that may be either generalized or localized to specific location. No sign of infection or trauma. Dyspareunia Vulvodynia
	Vestibular pain syndrome (also provoked vestibulodynia and vulvar vestibulitis)	Recurrent pain that is specifically elicited by pressure localized to the vulvar vestibule.
	Endometriosis	Recurrent pain associated with laparoscopically confirmed endometriosis
	Chronic pelvic pain syndrome	Cyclical pain localized to the pelvic region that is not associated with other gynaecological pain conditions.
	Dysmenorrhoea	Menstrual pain with no defined pathology. Diagnosis requires persistent pain that interferes with daily function
Gastrointestinal	Irritable bowel syndrome	Recurrent pain perceived in bowels without pathology. Preoccupation with bowel symptoms. Based on Rome III criteria
	Anal pain syndrome	Recurrent pain in the anus or anal canal without specific pathology. Unrelated to the need or process of defecation
Nervous	Pudendal neuralgia	Chronic pain in regions innervated by pudendal nerve. Pain with ischial palpation
Psychological/sexual	Genito-pelvic pain/penetration disorder	Persistent inability to achieve intercourse/penetration; pain with intercourse/penetration; fear or anxiety regarding pain or penetration; pelvic floor muscle abnormalities during attempted penetration. Causes significant distress/impairment
Musculoskeletal	Pelvic floor muscle pain syndrome	Recurrent pain in the pelvic floor. Associated with sexual and lower urinary tract symptoms. May have over activity or trigger points in pelvic floor
	Pelvic girdle pain	Pregnancy- or postpartum-related pain affecting any of the three pelvic joints. Problems with weight bearing and mobility
	Coccyx pain syndrome (Coccydynia)	Recurrent pain presenting in area of coccyx without signs of specific pathology

individuals who choose to continue being sexually active, can be quite high. An avoidance of sexual activity is a common response that can yield additional psychological and interpersonal conflict. Negative psychological responses to genito-pelvic pain may include increased pain-related anxiety and hypervigilance, as well as negative thoughts and feelings about one's sexual value and identity.

The extent of sexual interference may depend on whether pain is driven by physiological, psychological and/or interpersonal factors. Referring back to the UPOINT(S) approach, a number of physiological factors may produce pain that can become exquisitely intense during sexual activity. Furthermore, increased anxiety related to the expectation of pain may enhance pelvic muscle floor tension, which results in interference with penetration/vaginal spasms, secondary muscle pain and increased pressure against the organ(s) from which pain arises. Tenderness around the perineum, vulvovaginal area and/or the lower abdomen may further increase discomfort with physical contact. Finally, psychosocial factors shape how much an individual pays attention to this pain, as well

as how he or she responds to the pain (e.g. catastrophizing versus using distraction to reduce the pain experience).

Sexual dysfunction due to genito-pelvic pain is often an experience shared by the couple. In many cases, the partner directly contributes to the provocation of pain, as is the case with painful vaginal penetration or ejaculation, and this can create an environment of sexual ambivalence. The individual coping with pain may lose the motivation to engage in sexual activity, and his or her subsequent avoidance of sexual activity may encourage feelings of confusion and anger in the intimate partner. Understanding the couple's reaction to pain is paramount in determining its sexual impact: whereas some couples may immediately stop sexual activity when pain begins, other couples may learn to communicate about and pursue other sexually pleasurable activities that do not evoke pain.

Managing genito-pelvic pain

Women and men with genito-pelvic pain may seek help from a number of medical professionals in an attempt to understand and

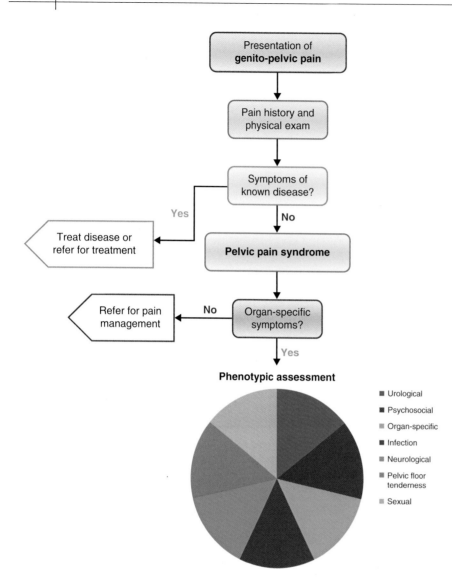

Figure 19.1 Pain assessment algorithm. A thorough pain history and physical exam are required to determine whether pain is idiopathic or due to a known disease. It is notable that treatments may fail to relieve pain and associated symptoms, and when no cause of pain can be found, a patient is considered to have an idiopathic pelvic pain syndrome. If no organ-specific symptoms are found, referrals for pain management may be made. When specific organs are implicated, it is recommended that a comprehensive phenotypic assessment be conducted to determine the respective contributions of urological/gynaecological, psychosocial, organ-specific, infectious, neurological, pelvic floor tenderness and sexual factors. Positive domains can further direct the referral and treatment process.

manage their pain. There are currently no clinically supported efficacious treatments for this family of idiopathic pain conditions. Topical treatments (e.g. corticosteroids, lidocaine and oestrogen for women) are often attempted first, as well as a course of oral antibiotics if infection is suspected to play a role. If urological symptoms are present, alpha blockers have been used, with equivocal results. Hormonal treatments in women, including use of oral contraceptives, may help reduce pain in a small subset of individuals. If these are unsuccessful, medical treatment for chronic pain may be given a trial such as an SSRI, TCA or gabapentin. In extreme cases, some individuals have sought the surgical excision of painful tissue to relieve pain.

Behavioural treatments are often attempted when biomedical treatments have failed. However, the optimal strategy is concurrent multidisciplinary treatment that focuses on pelvic floor rehabilitation and psychological/psychosexual pain management, as biomedical assessments and treatments are attempted. Pelvic floor physical therapy may facilitate pain reduction in individuals who present with pelvic floor muscle dysfunction. Notably, sustained pelvic pain may promote heightened pelvic floor tension, reduced muscle strength, and poor muscle control. Additionally, group and individual cognitive behavioural therapy for pelvic pain is designed to increase attention to sexual enjoyment and employ pain management strategies, such as mindfulness and distraction from pain. Behavioural approaches to pain management can provide individuals with the positive coping skills necessary to manage, and ideally accept, living with pain. Finally, couple therapy and/or sex therapy may be used to enhance communication about the impact of pain, as well as to focus on enhancing sexual motivation and arousal.

Table 19.3 UPOINT(S) classification assessment domains, symptoms and methods of evaluation

Domain	Symptoms	Evaluation
Urological	Painful urination Frequent urination Incomplete emptying Urgency	Residual volume > 100 ml Nocturia > 2/night Bothersome report
Psychosocial	Anxiety/fear of pain Pain catastrophizing Depression	Psych evaluation Validated questionnaires Fear/refusal of gynaecological exam
Organ specific	Pain localized to prostate or bladder	Rectal examination (prostate tenderness) Pre–post-prostate massage analysis Evidence of inflammation (leucocytosis, prostatic calcification, Hunner's ulcers) Bladder challenge test
Infection	Painful urination or ejaculation	Uropathogens (Gram-negative bacilli or Gram-positive Enterococcus) in mid stream urine or post-prostate massage
Neurological	Comorbid and/or related medical conditions	Irritable bowel syndrome, fibromyalgia, chronic fatigue syndrome, migraine headache, low back pain
	Sensitivity to heat, Pain with light touch, Pain when no stimulus is present	Patient report, sensory testing, conditioned pain modulation testing
Tenderness of pelvic floor	Pain when sitting for long periods, high stress	Abnormal findings in skeletal muscles of pelvic floor, palpable myofascial trigger points
Sexual dysfunction	Painful intercourse, erectile dysfunction, premature ejaculation, changes in desire/arousal	Patient report, validated questionnaires (IIEF or FSFI), painful gynaecological exam

IIEF, International Index of Erectile Function; FSFI, Female Sexual Functioning Index.

Further reading

Davis, S.N., Binik, Y.M. & Carrier, S. (2009) Sexual dysfunction and pelvic pain in men: a male sexual pain disorder? *Journal of Sex and Marital Therapy*, **35**, 182–205.

Dewitte, M., van Lankveld, J.V. & Crombez, G. (2011) Understanding sexual pain: a cognitive-motivational account. *Pain*, **152**, 251–253.

Nickel, J.C. & Shoskes, D. (2009) Phenotypic approach to the management of chronic prostatitis/chronic pelvic pain syndrome. *Current Urology Reports*, **10**, 307–312.

Rosenbaum, T.Y. (2007) Pelvic floor involvement in male and female sexual dysfunction and the role of pelvic floor rehabilitation in treatment: a literature review. *Journal of Sexual Medicine*, **4**, 4–13.

Van Lankveld, J.J.D.M., Granot, M., Weijmar Schultz, W.C.M. *et al.* (2010) Women's sexual pain disorders. *Journal of Sexual Medicine*, **7**, 615–631.

Wise, D. & Anderson, R. (2011) *A Headache in the Pelvis, a New Expanded 6th Edition: A New Understanding and Treatment for Chronic Pelvic Pain Syndromes*. National Center for Pelvic Pain Research, Occidental, CA.

CHAPTER 20

Ageing and Sexuality

Alison K. Wood[1] and Ross Runciman[2]

[1]Old Age Psychiatry, Sheffield, UK
[2]Wotton Lawn Hospital, Gloucester, UK

OVERVIEW

- Older people enjoy considerable sexual activity despite common preconceptions.

- Their sexual activity appears to be increasing as societal taboos lessen.

- Practical health issues, medication and polypharmacy can cause difficulties, but these can usually be overcome.

- Mental illnesses such as depression and dementia frequently adversely affect sexual activity.

- Older people frequently do not seek help for sexual difficulties and put problems down to old age but are usually willing to discuss this, if the subject is broached.

- Older people should be encouraged to seek help if their sexual life deteriorates and asked about sexual side effects of medication. Doctors' attitudes can hinder this process.

- LGBT people sometimes fear the loss of autonomy in old age and worry that they will re-experience the prejudices they often suffered in their youth.

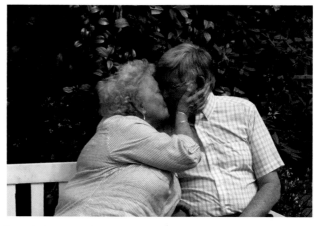

Figure 20.1 Your sexuality is part of the person you have always been. © 2014, Graham Hagan

The prevalence of sexual activity in older people

Elderly people often retain an interest in their sexual lives. This is becoming increasingly recognized, socially accepted and spoken about in mainstream media, through associations of retired people and online (Figure 20.1).

Recent evidence indicates that the prevalence of sexual activity amongst older people is increasing. This may be related to the loosening of societal taboos such as the increasing acceptability of sex outside marriage in many societies. In the future, online dating may also increase the opportunities to meet new partners despite the relative isolation of old age.

There are also indications that there may be an increasingly positive attitude to sexuality in later life and higher satisfaction with sexuality. Most elderly people consider sexual activity and associated feelings a natural part of later life. So, despite the prevalent belief amongst teenagers, sex does not end at 30 or even at 90 (Figure 20.2).

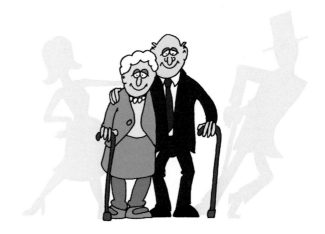

Figure 20.2 Despite the prevalent belief amongst teenagers, sex does not end at 30, or even at 90

Physical effects of ageing

For women, the biggest changes are associated with the climacteric which culminates in the menopause. Here, symptoms can involve itching of the vulva and of the vagina due to the decline in oestrogen

---

ABC of Sexual Health, Third Edition. Edited by Kevan Wylie.
© 2015 John Wiley & Sons, Ltd. Published 2015 by John Wiley & Sons, Ltd.

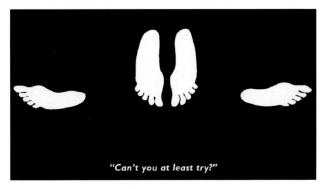

"Can't you at least try?"

Figure 20.3 Sex in old age can present a few challenges © 2014, Graham Hagan

Women	Men
Climacteric and menopause	Low testosterone
Gynaecology problems: prolapse, dry vagina	Penis problems: erectile dysfunction
Urological problems: incontinence	Prostate problems: incontinence and retention
Diabetes and its consequences such as neuropathy and infections (e.g. candidiasis) Cardiovascular disease: myocardial infarction, heart failure, ischaemic heart disease, hypertension Neurological illness: such as Parkinson's disease Arthritis and osteoporosis	

Figure 20.4 Physical effects of illness and ageing factors affecting sexual dysfunction

levels, associated with the waning function of the ovaries. However, these symptoms probably affect the sex lives of only a minority of women. For men, there is no direct analogue to the menopause, although there is growing evidence that men's testosterone levels reduce with age. This decline is much slower than that of oestrogen in women; yet there could be an association with more difficulty producing firm, long-duration erections and with reaching orgasm. However, the most significant difficulties with ageing and sexual function are not associated with the direct physiological changes, but rather with the psychological and societal impacts of getting older. There is a toxic combination of the predominance of youthful images of sex in society, plus for some people the nihilism of sex where reproduction is impossible and the inter-related self-perception of declining attractiveness with age, the latter being especially prevalent in women (Figure 20.3).

Physical effects of illness

Biological age does not automatically lead to more sexual dysfunction for either gender, apart from men's erectile and orgasmic problems. Furthermore, the link between poor health and sexual dysfunction may be more related to mental, rather than physical health problems.

However, it has been found that there is a consistent association between good physical health and higher levels of sexual activity in the elderly, in various American surveys. Many common diseases and health conditions have limited impact on sexual performance. Certain diseases do recurrently cause sexual dysfunction, most prominently, diabetes. Across American, European and Australian surveys, this increasingly common disease had significant negative effects on sexual activity in men and women; with females experiencing reduced sexual activity, men experiencing increased erectile dysfunction and less frequent masturbation for both sexes.

Previous health problems have also been noted to contribute to sexual dysfunction in older life, for example women with a history of sexually transmitted infections (STIs), appear to increase their chances of reporting dyspareunia and their likelihood of experiencing lubrication problems in later life. This could be a worrying trend for our future older adults, with the recent increase in rates of STIs (Figure 20.4).

Effects of psychiatric illness including dementia

Arguably, the biggest impact health has on sexual dysfunction is from mental health. This is actually a broad spectrum, ranging from the more psychological perceptions of couples, whereby those most satisfied in their relationships experience subjectively better sex, to more diagnosable illness, mainly depression and dementia. There is circumstantial evidence that psychological stressors, that are perhaps more common in later life, affect sexual performance, such as losing a loved one and being a carer for an ill family member.

Depression is a common disease in the elderly and has been associated with decreased sexual function and increased anorgasmia in both sexes, with women gaining less pleasure from sex and men encountering more erectile dysfunction. Dementia is a growing mental health problem which poses difficult ethical dilemmas and practical issues for couples who wish to continue their sex lives. Previously a taboo subject, key charities and support groups are encouraging debate and discussions about this as well as offering support, such as the UK-based Alzheimer's Society. They highlight how sex and physical intimacy can be important for couples in which one of them has a diagnosis of dementia. However, those with the disease are unpredictable in their response and consent can become a difficult issue.

Effects of drugs and polypharmacy

Older people tend to take more medications, and multiple medications or polypharmacy have effects which are difficult to predict. Anticoagulants, cardiovascular medications, those used to control hypertension and cholesterol have been associated with lower sexual desire and frequency of sex.

More generally, there is evidence for many drugs impacting sexual function across all adult age groups. Antidepressants are a well-known source of sexual dysfunction, selective serotonin reuptake inhibitors (SSRIs), often first-line treatment in depression, can cause loss of sexual interest, anorgasmia and erectile dysfunction. Tricyclic antidepressants, used as second-line drugs for depression or in lower doses for chronic pain, can cause anorgasmia in men and women.

Other drugs used to treat conditions more common in the elderly can change sexual function in unpredictable ways. Benzodiazepines, sometimes given to aid sleep in small doses or for short-term management of behavioural aspects of dementia, can initially reduce desire, but later increase libido as they can be disinhibiting. Equally L-dopa, used to treat Parkinson's disease, can cause hypersexuality.

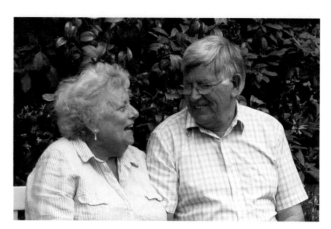

Figure 20.5 With appropriate help, people can enjoy physical intimacy at any age.

Social effects of ageing

Several studies have concluded that one of the most significant factors limiting sexuality in old age is the lack of a partner. Another important issue can be the impact of older adult accommodation. Sexuality is not always considered as important within a residential home environment, where privacy can be very difficult to obtain and where couples with different nursing needs may even be housed apart. Specific difficulties arise for older lesbian, gay, bisexual or transsexual (LGBT) people, some of whom fear greatly the prospect of an old age in a potentially unsympathetic or even critical, mainstream environment. However, attitudes are changing, for example gay marriage is now legal in the UK.

Help-seeking behaviour

Help is available for sexual difficulties in old age but people often do not approach services. Some studies have shown that many people believe that sexual difficulties are a normal part of old age and do not cause much distress. Such recent work has highlighted that often difficulties were not considered to be serious and were frequently just left to see whether they would get better spontaneously. Many did not view sexual functioning as a medical issue at all, more as a recreational pursuit about which it may not be appropriate to consult a doctor. Some patients were aware that the doctor might be uncomfortable with the subject of sex themselves and some older people even feared disapproval, especially from a younger doctor, regarding their sexual activity.

The relevance of education for health professionals

The perceived attitude of the health professional, who is approached, clearly affects help-seeking behaviour. It has been shown that doctors are more likely to broach the subject of sexual functioning with younger patients than older patients and that cultural factors can have a great bearing on the attitudes of both doctors and patients, creating barriers to effective communication. Also, behaviours in different countries can vary considerably.

Conclusions

There are barriers to sexual activity in old age. Changes due to ageing, illness, medication use, social circumstances and residential environment can all be a hindrance. However, emphatically, age is no bar to treatment. The increasing social acceptability of discussions about sexuality in old age, the availability of anonymous advice online and improved medical education should all help to facilitate the freedom and capacity to enjoy our sexuality into old age (Figure 20.5).

Further reading

Alzheimer's Society. (2014) Sex and Dementia. Website link: http://www.alzheimers.org.uk/site/scripts/documents_info.php?documentID=129 Accessed on 15/05/2013

American Association of Retired Persons (1999) *AARP/Modern Maturity Sexuality Study*. Author, Washington, DC.

American Association of Retired Persons (2010) *Sex, Romance, and Relationships: AARP Survey of Midlife and Older Adults (Publication No, D19234)*. Author, Washington, DC.

Aubin, S. & Heiman, J. (2004) Sexual dysfunction from a relationship perspective. In: Harvey, J., Wenzel, A. & Sprecher, S. (eds), *The Handbook of Sexuality in Close Relationships*. Lawrence Erlbaum Associates, Inc., Mahwah, NJ, pp. 477–519.

Beckman, N., Waern, M., Gustafson, D. & Skoog, I. (2008) Secular trends in self reported sexual activity and satisfaction in Swedish 70 year olds: a cross sectional survey of four populations, 1971–2001. *BMJ*, **337** (**7662**), 151–154.

Brody, S. (2010) The relative health benefits of different sexual activities. *Journal of Sexual Medicine*, **7**, 1336–1361.

Burgess, E.O. (2004) Sexuality in midlife and later life couples. In: Harvey, J., Wenzel, A. & Sprecher, S. (eds), *The Handbook of Sexuality in Close Relationships*. Lawrence Erlbaum Associates, Inc., Mahwah, NJ, pp. 437–454.

DeLamater, J. (2012) Sexual expression in later life: a review and synthesis. *Journal of Sex Research*, **49**, 125–141.

Hinchliff, S. & Gott, M. (2011) Seeking medical help for sexual concerns in mid- and later life: a review of the literature. *Journal of Sex Research*, **48**, 106–117.

Hyde, Z., Flicker, L., Hankey, G.J. *et al.* (2010) Prevalence of sexual activity and associated factors in men aged 75 to 95 years: a cohort study. *Annals of Internal Medicine*, **153** (**11**), 693–702.

Krychman, M. (2007) Vaginal atrophy: the 21st century health issue affecting quality of life. Medscape Ob/Gyn & Women's Health. Retrieved from http://www.medscape.com/viewarticle/561934 Accessed on 04/12/2014.

Laumann, E.O., Das, A. & Waite, L.J. (2008) Sexual dysfunction among older adults: prevalence and risk factors from a Nationally Representative U.S. probability sample of men and women 57–85 years of age. *Journal of Sexual Medicine*, **5** (**10**), 2300–2311.

Lindau, S.T., Schumm, L.P., Laumann, E.O., Levinson, W., O'Muircheartaigh, C. & Waite, L. (2007) A study of sexuality and health among older adults in the United States. *New England Journal of Medicine*, **357**, 762–774.

Schindel, A.W., Ando, K.A., Nelson, C.J. *et al* (2010) Medical student sexuality: how sexual experience and sexuality training impact U.S. and Canadian medical students' comfort in dealing with patients' sexuality in clinical practice. *Academic Medicine*, **85**, 1321–1330.

Smith, S. (2007) Drugs that cause sexual dysfunction. *Psychiatry*, **6** (**3**), 111–114.

Waite, L.J., Laumann, E.O., Levinson, W. *et al.* (2010) *National Social Life, Health, and Aging Project (NSHAP). ICPSR20541-v5*. Inter-University Consortium for Political and Social Research [distributor], Ann Arbor, MI.

Wood, A., Runciman, R., Wylie, K.R. & McManus, R. (2012) An update on female sexual function and dysfunction in old age and its relevance to old age psychiatry. *Aging and Disease*, **3** (**5**), 373–84.

CHAPTER 21

Paraphilia Behaviour and Disorders

Kevan Wylie

World Association for Sexual Health, Sheffield, UK

OVERVIEW

- Paraphilic behaviours such as fetishistic behaviour is commonly practised in the community
- Paraphilic behaviours are often unrelated to paraphilic disorders
- Certain paraphilic disorders may lead to conflict with society and imprisonment
- Pharmacological, endocrinological and psychotherapeutic options are effective for certain paraphilic disorders

The paraphilias or sexual preference disorders as listed in the ICD-10 (F65) are a group of preferences that were considered out with normality. With increasing acceptance of diversity, many of the conditions historically described as 'perversions' are no longer considered such within the DSM-5 and will probably be removed in the forthcoming revision for the ICD-11. Although paraphilias have not disappeared from the DSM-5, there is an attempt to clearly distinguish between the behaviour itself (i.e. sexual masochism) and a disorder stemming from that behaviour (i.e. sexual masochism disorder). To differentiate between atypical sexual interest and a mental disorder, DSM-5 requires that, for diagnosis, people with such interests exhibit the following: (i) feel personal distress about their interest, not merely distress resulting from society's disapproval; or (ii) have a sexual desire or behaviour that involves another person's psychological distress, injury, or death or a desire for sexual behaviours involving unwilling persons or persons unable to give legal consent.

Fetishistic behaviour

A fetish is an inanimate object or non-genital or breast body part that a person must focus on to become sexually aroused and in extreme cases to achieve sexual satisfaction. The reliance on some non-living object as a stimulus for arousal and sexual gratification may arise for a number of reasons. However for many people there is experimentation with fetishist behaviour, which is not a fetish

by definition. The feet and toes (podophilia) was by far the most common sexual preference for body parts or features in a recent study. Likewise, footwear and objects worn on legs and buttocks including stockings and skirts were the sexual preferences for objects associated with the body. Promiscuity became unfashionable with the rise of sexually transmitted infections, including HIV and many couples were looking at ways to keep their sex lives fresh. Historically, psychoanalysts believe that severe castration anxiety and denial that the female does not have a phallus leads to the fetish object representing magical substitution for the female's absent phallus or that the fetish object represents an important parental type individual who has in the fetishists' earlier life humiliated him. In the latter case the individual dehumanizes the other person and substitutes them with an inanimate fetish object, the consequence is an act of cruelty and triumph. However, others describe learnt behaviour resulting from conditioned sexual response to specific stimuli as the reason for development of a fetish.

A recent development – CMNM (Clothed Male Naked Male) – is a fetish about exhibitionism and voyeurism and is practiced by men who like to be naked in front of dressed men or by dressed men who like to look at and be in the presence of naked men. It has been argued that nudity and exposure of body parts and the genitals allows communication of affection and friendship intimacy, but also expression of power and control to show emotions that cannot be spoken by men. The interface with social conscience issues such as naked bike rides and sexual activity in public places – PSE (Public Sex Environment) – again demonstrates increasing changes of societal acceptance.

Variations of fetishism include the use of body jewellery, piercings, commonly the Prince Albert, and tattoos. The Prince Albert piercing is a ring-style piercing that extends along the underside of the glans from the urethral opening to where the glans meets the shaft of the penis. Making changes to one's body parts can progress in more severe cases to the Skoptic syndrome, in which a person is preoccupied with or engages in genital self-mutilation such as castration, penectomy or clitoridectomy. This may form the basis of the sexual fantasy for masturbation.

Fetishistic transvestism is where articles of clothing are worn to create the appearance of a person of the opposite sex, almost always a male dressing as a female, and using hair pieces and make up with sexual arousal and sexual activity thereafter. There is almost always a strong desire to remove clothing after orgasm. This is differentiated from transgender conditions and gender dysphoria (see Chapter 26).

Sadomasochistic behaviour

This is the preference for sexual activity that involves bondage or the infliction of pain or humiliation. Examples include face slapping, flagellation, use of gags, knives or verbal humiliation. When the individual prefers to be the recipient of such stimulation, it is termed masochism. Recent studies have suggested that 'BDSM' (commonly known as a synthesis of bondage and discipline, dominance and submission and sadomasochism) may be more a sexual interest or subculture attractive to a minority of people and for most participants should not be seen as a pathological symptom of past abuse or difficulty with normal sex. This is discussed further in Chapter 25.

The DSM-5 differentiation between the paraphilias and paraphilic disorders has been a decisive step forward in depathologizing consenting adults who engage in diverse sexual behaviours (see Box 21.1).

Exhibitionistic, frotteuristic and voyeuristic behaviour

These conditions are commonly considered courtship disorders with exhibitionism describing sexual arousal by exposing ones' genitals to unsuspecting strangers, typically in inappropriate settings and usually men towards women. Voyeurism, the 'peeping tom', involves sexual arousal by observing nude individuals without their knowledge or consent. In both cases there are often intense urges and recurrent behaviour even though it may be ego dystonic once orgasm has occurred. Frotteurism is sexual arousal by rubbing ones' genitals against others in public. These offences may lead to conviction and indictment to imprisonment for a term not exceeding 2 years under the UK Sexual Offences Act, 2003. Recent studies suggest that respondents report either exhibitionistic or voyeuristic behaviour would be entertained by a significant minority on the basis that they would not be caught. In the latter study, respondents were also significantly more likely to engage in other

---

Box 21.1

'It is National Coalition for Sexual Freedom (NCSF's) opinion that the revised DSM-5 criteria have been successful in changing the way BDSM behaviour by a parent is considered during a child custody hearing, thereby removing BDSM behaviour as a detrimental factor in those cases. NCSF is grateful on behalf of its constituents that the American Psychiatric Association, in particular the Sexual and gender Identity Disorders Workgroup and the Paraphilias sub-workgroup, responded to the evidence of discrimination against consenting adults who engage in unusual sexual practices and revised the criteria and text in the DSM-5 to ensure that these individuals are no longer being misdiagnosed with mental disorder and denied child custody based on that misdiagnosis'.

---

paraphilic-like behaviour, namely sadomasochistic behaviour and transvestic fetishist behaviour.

Paedophilia and further behaviour attracting forensic attention

Paedophilia is a sexual preference for children, usually pre-pubertal. The Sexual Offences Act, 2003 allows for conviction on indictment to imprisonment for a term of up to 14 years for arranging or facilitating child prostitution or pornography. A number of studies have attempted to identify differences in the neurobiological structure of paedophilic offenders. Recent findings suggest specific impaired neural networks relating to phenotypic characteristics might account for the heterogeneous results identified with neuro-imaging studies and that these neuro-anatomical abnormalities may be a dimensional rather than a categorical nature supporting the notion of a multifaceted disorder.

Other conditions involving non-consenting participants include intercourse with an animal (bestiality, or zoophilia) and with corpses (necrophilia). A commonly cited internet source, the 'deviant desires' website has a manifesto that any sexual **fantasy** is acceptable and that nothing is sacred and beyond sexualization, but that sexual interactions must be 'safe, sane and consensual'.

Problematic hypersexual behaviour

This is a clinical syndrome characterized by loss of control over sexual fantasies, urges and behaviours which are accompanied by adverse consequences and/or personal distress. Some have used the term 'sex addiction' and there is general agreement that the essential features include impaired control and continuation of behaviour despite consequences. Types of hypersexual behaviour include masturbation, use of pornography, sexual behaviour with consenting adults including solicitation of sex workers, cybersex, telephone sex and strip clubs. Cybersex is the inability to freely choose to stop use of the internet for sexual arousal and pleasure and continuing behaviour despite adverse consequences.

It is unclear why this syndrome occurs, but it is usually multi-factorial with developmental factors including problems with attachment and feeling neglected allowing sex to become a temporary close relationship that feels good. Cognitive markers are poor self-worth, self-esteem and negative emotions; neurobiological substrates, biological vulnerability, disinhibition of sexual excitation and cultural influences (as societal norms). Depression and other co-morbid mental health issues and narcissistic personality traits are relatively common findings. Several models have been described including the impulsive compulsive model (which is normophilic and not paraphilic) and the addictive model. The definition of such a disorder is controversial and whilst advocates have proposed this is a discrete condition, it did not emerge in the new DSM-5. This is discussed further in Chapter 22. Hypersexuality does occur in certain neurological conditions including Parkinson's disease, particularly when on dopa medication, brain injury and dementia.

The Klüver–Bucy syndrome is a rare situation with hypersexuality, hyperorality, hyperphagia and hyperdocility.

Therapeutic options

Interventions include pharmacological suppression of androgens, the use of cyproterone, selective serotonin re-uptake inhibitors (SSRIs), GnRH analogues, naloxone and in some countries medroxyprogesterone that acts like testosterone in exerting negative feedback on the hypothalamo-pituitary axis.

Psychological interventions include covert sensitization with the linking of paraphilic behaviour to a fantasy of an aversive stimulus (such as being before a magistrate or court judge); orgasmic reconditioning pairing culturally appropriate imagery with orgasmic pleasure; cognitive restructuring; social skills training and victim empathy. Aversion therapy is rarely part of clinical care.

Other psychological interventions include treatment of co-morbidities (axis 1 and axis 2) and the 12-step treatment for sexual addiction that may be offered as group or residential treatment. Individual therapies include emotional focused therapy, cognitive therapy, psychodynamic therapy and couples and systemic therapy.

Conclusions

Many paraphilic preferences and behaviour have been declassified as a clinical disorder and do not cause any personal distress to an individual or couple relationship. There is often co-morbidity of behaviours and most individuals do not seek medical assistance.

Further reading

American Psychiatric Association (APA) (2000) *Diagnostic and Statistical Manual of Mental Disorders DSM-5*. APA, Washington, DC.

Binet, A. (1887) Le fétichisme dans l'amour. *Revue Philosophique*, **24**, 143–152.

Carnes, P.J., Delmonico, D.L., Griffin, E. & Moriarity, J. (2001) *In the Shadows of the Net: Breaking Free of Online Compulsive Sexual Behavior*. Hazelden Educational Materials, Center City, MN.

Freud, S. (1940) Splitting of the ego in the process of defence. *Standard edition*, **23**, 275–278.

Griffiths, M.D. (2012) Internet sex addiction: a review of empirical research. *Addiction Research & Theory*, **20** (2), 111–124.

Hall, P. (2011) A biopsychosocial view of sex addiction. *Sexual and Relationship Therapy*, **26** (3), 217–228.

Kafka, M.P. (2010) Hypersexual disorder: a proposed diagnosis for DSM-V. *Archives of Sexual Behavior*, **39** (2), 377–400.

Kaplan, M.S. & Krueger, R.B. (2010) Diagnosis, assessment, and treatment of hypersexuality. *Journal of Sex Research*, **47** (2-3), 181–198.

Marshall, L.E. & Briken, P. (2010) Assessment, diagnosis, and management of hypersexual disorders. *Current Opinion in Psychiatry*, **23** (6), 570–573.

Marshall, L.E. & Marshall, W.L. (2006) Sexual addiction in incarcerated sexual offenders. *Sexual Addiction & Compulsivity*, **13** (4), 377–390.

McManus, M.A., Hargreaves, P., Rainbow, L., & Alison, L.J. (2013). Paraphilias: definition, diagnosis and treatment. F1000prime reports, 5, 36.

Niklas Långström, M.D. (2006) High rates of sexual behavior in the general population: correlates and predictors. *Archives of Sexual Behavior*, **35** (1), 37–52.

Nordling, N., Sandnabba, N.K. & Santtila, P. (2000) The prevalence and effects of self-reported childhood sexual abuse among sadomasochistically oriented males and females. *Journal of Child Sexual Abuse*, **9** (1), 53–63.

Poeppl, T.B., Nitschke, J., Santtila, P. et al. (2013) Association between brain structure and phenotypic characteristics in pedophilia. *Journal of Psychiatric Research*, **47** (5), 678–685.

Richters, J., De Visser, R.O., Rissel, C.E., Grulich, A.E. & Smith, A. (2008) Demographic and psychosocial features of participants in bondage and discipline, "sadomasochism" or dominance and submission (BDSM): Data from a national survey. *Journal of Sexual Medicine*, **5** (7), 1660–1668.

Rye, B.J. & Meaney, G.J. (2007) Voyeurism: it is good as long as we do not get caught. *International Journal of Sexual Health*, **19** (1), 47–56.

Sagarin, B.J., Cutler, B., Cutler, N., Lawler-Sagarin, K.A. & Matuszewich, L. (2009) Hormonal changes and couple bonding in consensual sadomasochistic activity. *Archives of Sexual Behavior*, **38** (2), 186–200.

Scorolli, C., Ghirlanda, S., Enquist, M., Zattoni, S. & Jannini, E.A. (2007) Relative prevalence of different fetishes. *International Journal of Impotence Research*, **19** (4), 432–437.

Stoller, R.J. (1979) Centerfold: an essay on excitement. *Archives of General Psychiatry*, **36** (9), 1019.

Wright, S. (2014) Kinky parents and child custody: the effect of the DSM-5 differentiation between the paraphilias and paraphilix disorders. *Archives of Sexual Behaviours*, **43** (7), 1257–1258., ahead of print.

CHAPTER 22

Impulsive/Compulsive Sexual Behaviour

Eli Coleman

Program in Human Sexuality, University of Minnesota, MN, USA

> **OVERVIEW**
>
> - Clinicians will often encounter individuals with impulsive and/or compulsive sexual behaviour. There is growing recognition that this behaviour can be pathological
> - There is no universal consensus on what to call this syndrome, the diagnostic criteria or the methods to treat it
> - Careful assessment and multimodal/multidisciplinary treatment can offer assistance to many individuals suffering from ICSB
> - There is still much to learn about this syndrome. Specialists are needed in assessment and treatment, and clinicians need to keep up with emerging literature in order to provide the best evidence-based care.

One of the common sexual health problems clinicians will encounter is normative (normophilic) sexual behaviour that is impulsive and/or compulsive. While most clinicians are familiar with sexual dysfunctions and paraphilias, less is known about this type of sexual problem. This chapter will attempt to fill that gap in knowledge with the caveat that there is still a dearth of research, understanding and consensus on nomenclature, aetiology and treatment approaches. This chapter will limit itself to normophilic impulsive/compulsive sexual behaviour (ICSB) and refer the reader to Chapter 21 on paraphilias for a discussion of those types of problems.

Despite disagreements within the field, there is growing recognition among clinicians that sexual behaviour can become pathologically impulsive and/or compulsive. It is not unusual for normal sexual behaviour to be at times impulsive, compulsive, driven and distracting which is pleasurable and satisfying. The question becomes when does it become overly so and the person is in need of psychological or psychiatric treatment. There is intense debate about this and there is no universally accepted clinical criterion or assessment tool to aid the clinician in making this assessment.

In the meantime, the problem exists and people are suffering. So, with caution, the clinician can be guided by the extant knowledge regarding proposed clinical criteria and treatment approaches that have been explicated. They can also consult colleagues who have

more experience in working with this clinical population or refer their patients to them.

What do we call it?

This clinical phenomenon has been described with a variety of terms in the literature: *hypersexuality, hyperphilia, erotomania, satyriasis, promiscuity, Don Juanism, Don Juanitaism*, and, more recently, *sexual addiction, compulsive sexual behaviour* and *paraphilia-related disorder*. In the International Classification of Diseases (ICD) (Version 10), there is a category of *Excessive Sexual Drive*. Examples of this are *nymphomania* and *satyriasis*. At present, the ICD-11 is being prepared and this category is undergoing scrutiny but it is unclear what the outcome will be.

The American Psychiatric Association (APA) has entered this debate and most recently the committee assigned to recommend revisions to the current Diagnostic and Statistical Manual (DSM-5) had suggested the term and a new category of sexual disorders: *hypersexual disorder*. However, the APA did not accept this proposal and even removed the example of a *Sexual Disorder Not Otherwise Specified*. Currently, there is no appropriate category within the sexual disorders section that seems to fit what clinicians see as ICSB. The best alternative seems to be to use *Impulse Control Not Otherwise Specified*.

In my work and throughout this chapter, I use the term *impulsive/compulsive sexual behaviour* to describe this syndrome. There are two different types of ICSB: paraphilic and non-paraphilic. In many ways, they are similar. The main difference is that one involves normative sexual behaviour and the other involves socially anomalous behaviour or that which is considered deviant. However, as stated previously, I will limit my discussion in this chapter to the non-paraphilic types.

I have chosen this term in order to be simply descriptive and to recognize the multiple pathological pathways and treatments. We have seen patients with more of an impulsive type pattern; a compulsive type pattern or something mixed. This term is limiting as well because it sometimes is best characterized as a function of a personality disorder rather than an impulse or compulsive drive. While I recognize the limitation and the fact that is not a facile term, it challenges the clinician to think the clinical syndrome through and try to understand its dynamics and as a result develop an individualized treatment approach.

ABC of Sexual Health, Third Edition. Edited by Kevan Wylie.
© 2015 John Wiley & Sons, Ltd. Published 2015 by John Wiley & Sons, Ltd.

For purposes of operationalizing my definition, I have described ICSB as putative clinical syndrome characterized by the experience of sexual urges, sexually arousing fantasies and sexual behaviours that are recurrent, intense and cause distressful interference in one's daily life.

Non-paraphilic ICSB

As stated previously non-paraphilic ICSB are similar to the paraphilias but they involve normative and conventional sexual behaviour that is engaged in recurrently and intensely, yet with similar negative consequences and distress. The APA has debated the inclusion of a new clinical category to describe this clinical syndrome. There was a proposal to create a new category of sexual disorders: *hypersexual disorder*. There had been a category of *Sexual Disorder Not Otherwise Specified* which included an example of *Don Juanism* ('distress about a pattern of repeated sexual relationships involving a succession of lovers who are experienced by the individual only as things to be used' in *DSM III, III-R, IV, IV TR*). However, the APA did not accept this proposal and even removed the example of *Sexual Disorder Not Otherwise Specified*. Currently, there is no appropriate category within the sexual disorders section that seems to fit what clinicians see as ICSB. The best alternative seems to be to use *Impulse Control Not Otherwise Specified*.

There was also consideration of including this clinical phenomenon under a proposed new category of *Behavioural Addictions*. However, this was not accepted either. The category of *Behavioural Addictions* was added but it only includes pathological gambling as one of the categories.

Clinicians will need to follow this debate, and it is uncertain how this clinical syndrome will be classified in the revisions of the DSM and/or ICD. This issue needs to be resolved.

The proposed category of *Hypersexual Disorder* at least recognized the various potential pathological pathways but the term still connotes that the behaviour may be 'excessive' (which can be quite subjective and fail to recognize the wide range of normal sexual drive) or conveys the notion that the behaviour is driven by hypersexual drive. As a basic appetitive drive, sex could be deregulated in a hyper or hypo state. We seem to have no qualms about diagnosing hypersexual desire disorder but it becomes more difficult to find consensus about hypersexual drive dysregulation. There are many problems with the hyposexual desire notion as well.

The major problem with the category of *Behavioural Addictions* is that it assumes that it has commonalities in clinical expression, aetiology, comorbidity, physiology and treatment with *Substance Use Disorders*. This may be one type of pathway or similarity but probably a narrow way of viewing the vast majority with this clinical syndrome. The problems of this approach have been articulated by many although there are many who are very comfortable with this approach. The public, too, seem to find the notion of *sexual addiction* to be easily understood. I have argued elsewhere and repeatedly that this is a misnomer and at best can be used metaphorically. However, the term obviates the complexity and the multiple pathways that this clinical syndrome can manifest.

There is no consensus on the types of non-paraphilic ICSB. There are at least seven subtypes: compulsive cruising and multiple partners, compulsive fixation on an unattainable partner, compulsive autoeroticism (masturbation), compulsive use of erotica, compulsive use of the Internet for sexual purposes, compulsive multiple love relationships and compulsive sexuality in a relationship. The type of sexual behaviour (including fantasy) can vary but the dynamics of impulsivity or compulsivity are very similar.

The danger of overpathologizing this disorder

The overpathologizing of sexual behaviour (including ICSB) can occur by failing to recognize the wide range of normal human sexual expression – not only in frequency but also in variety. It can also occur among clinicians who have overly conservative attitudes and values regarding human sexual expression. It is important for professionals to be comfortable with a wide range of normal sexual behaviour – both in type and in frequency. Another problem can be caused by lack of knowledge and training. Many clinicians lack appropriate training in human sexuality. As in evaluating any condition outside of one's area of expertise, it is good practice to seek consultation from a specialist in treating sexual disorders.

Sometimes individuals, with their own restrictive values, will diagnose themselves with ICSB, thus creating their own distress. Therefore, it is very important to distinguish between an individual whose values conflict with his or her sexual behaviour and one who engages in sexual behaviours that are driven by impulsive, obsessive and/or compulsive mechanisms.

It is very important to distinguish ICSB from individuals who are in a conflict with their own values or those of their relationships or society. It is very important to distinguish problems that are a function of interpersonal conflict – usually a difference in values; or, to be careful to distinguish different levels of sexual desire within a couple. Many couples are simply desire-discrepant. The same trap exists for diagnosing someone with less desire with hypoactive sexual desire to someone who has higher sexual desire and assuming that they are drive-dysregulated.

Also it is important to distinguish between something that is a problem versus ICSB. Many people develop problems related to their sexual behaviour. Sometimes there is a knee-jerk reaction to labelling the problem as a function of a pathological state. I have found that it is very helpful to view sexual behaviours on a continuum. At one end of the continuum is healthy sexuality; at the other end is the clinical syndrome of ICSB (see Figure 22.1).

It is also helpful to distinguish between sexual behaviour that might better be understood from a developmental perspective versus that of a pathological condition. Sexual behaviour in adolescents can often appear as impulsive or compulsive. The development context should always be considered.

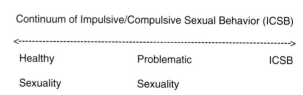

Figure 22.1 Continuum of ICSB.

Treatment

Treatment of ICSB usually involves a combination of psycho- and pharmacotherapies. One should always consider that many problematic behaviours are just that and many of these problems can respond to brief treatment and psychoeducation. If that fails, or it is clear that the problem is more serious, it is more likely that a course of psychotherapy will be needed, often with adjunct pharmacotherapy. The psychological and pharmacological treatment is described elsewhere. A first step is getting control of the behaviour but the treatment does not end there. Once ICSB is under control, the patient is ready to learn new intimacy skills and develop healthy sexual functioning. This may involve major shifts in the ways in which patients interact with other people, are intimate with their partner, or approach sexual activity with themselves or with a partner. These are learned skills. Patients need guidance from the therapist on ways of improving their relationship skills and approaching sexual activity. The basic principles of sex therapy can be very useful in this stage of the therapeutic process.

Repairing a broken relationship comes at a later stage of the therapeutic process when the ICSB is under control, new patterns of relating can be learned, and trust restored.

We have found that many of our patients benefit from ongoing psychotherapeutic support through a much less intensive but ongoing therapy. The bottom line is that most patients need some type of ongoing support to maintain their progress and to grow further as sexual beings. Because ICSB is a deep-seated psychosexual disorder, a long process is needed not only to gain control over it but also to consolidate long-term gains and prevent relapse. The ultimate goal is not just to gain control over dysfunctional sexual behaviours but also to assist individuals to find healthy and pleasurable means of sexual expression and intimacy functioning.

Pharmacological treatment

Pharmacological treatment has been shown to be an effective adjunct to the psychological treatment of ICSB. It takes a trained clinician who is familiar with these medications and the literature to effectively utilize these medications in treating patients with ICSB. We need controlled clinical trials in order to develop a more evidence-based clinical approach to the pharmacological treatment of ICSB. However, there is at least some evidence that a number of helpful treatment options are available. Clinicians should keep abreast of the literature for future developments, as this is still an emerging field of study.

Conclusion

ICSB is a serious clinical disorder that deserves attention from health care professionals. It can be easily overlooked and yet can lead to serious distress and negative consequences. The difficulty of identifying this problem is compounded by the fact that we do not have a consensus on what to call this syndrome, the diagnostic criteria or the methods to treat it. We rely on a case report literature for guidance in the absence of clinical trials of psychological or pharmacological treatment. Careful assessment and combined multimodal and multidisciplinary treatment can offer assistance to many individuals suffering from ICSB. Specialists are needed in assessment and treatment.

There is much to be learned about this syndrome. Clinicians will need to keep up with the emerging literature in order to provide the best evidence-based care. In the meantime, it is encouraging that we have found effective treatments that can offer hope for improved sexual and intimate lives for patients who suffer from ICSB.

Further reading

American Psychiatric Association (2013) *Diagnostic and Statistical Manual of Mental Disorders*, 5th edn. American Psychiatric Publishing, Arlington, VA.

Bradford, J. (2000) Treatment of sexual deviation using a pharmacologic approach. *Journal of Sex Research*, **37** (**3**), 248–257.

Carnes, P. (1983) *Out of the Shadows: Understanding Sexual Addiction*. CompCare Publishers, Minneapolis, MN.

Coleman, E. (1991) Compulsive sexual behavior: New concepts and treatments. *Journal of Psychology and Human Sexuality*, **4**, 37–52.

Coleman, E. (1995) Treatment of compulsive sexual behavior. In: Rosen, R.C. & Leiblum, S.R. (eds), *Case Studies in Sex Therapy*. Guilford Press, New York, pp. 333–349.

Coleman, E. (2011) Impulsive/compulsive sexual behavior: assessment and treatment. In: Grant, J.E. & Potenza, M.N. (eds), *The Oxford Handbook of Impulse Control Disorders*. Oxford University Press, New York.

Kafka, M.P. (2009) Hypersexual disorder: a proposed diagnosis for DSM-V. *Archives of Sexual Behavior*, **39**, 377–400.

Money, J. (1986) *Lovemaps: Clinical Concepts of Sexual/Erotic Health and Pathology, Paraphilia, and Gender Transposition in Childhood, Adolescence, and Maturity*. Irvington, New York.

CHAPTER 23

Forensic Sexology

Don Grubin[1,2]

[1]Institute of Neuroscience, Newcastle University, Newcastle upon Tyne, UK
[2]Northumberland Tyne and Wear NHS Foundation Trust, Newcastle upon Tyne, UK

OVERVIEW

- High sex drive, sexual preoccupation and emotional dysregulation are potential areas for medical intervention in sex offenders
- Testosterone, serotonin and dopamine are particularly important influences on sexual arousal and sex drive
- Mood stabilizers, SSRIs and antiandrogens may help in the management of problematic sexual behaviour
- Treatment algorithms based on a combination of risk and medical indication can help in prescribing decisions
- Doctors can treat sex offender patients without becoming agents of 'social control'.

Introduction

Most sex offenders are capable of controlling their behaviour, they just choose not to do so. Like any criminal, they are typically dealt with by the criminal justice system rather than by doctors. In some cases, however, there may be pressure on doctors to detain offenders in hospital or to medicate them (what the media likes to refer to as chemical castration). But doctors treat patients for medical indications, they are not 'agents of social control'; patient welfare, not risk management, is the basis of medical practice. It is therefore important for doctors to be able to differentiate those individuals for whom they can provide genuine benefit from those where they are asked to perform non-medical roles.

The focus of sex offender treatment is generally psychologically based. For some individuals, however, sex drive can be so strong or sexual preoccupation so dominant, that psychological therapy on its own is not viable. No matter how 'psychological' sex offending may be, it is dependent on sex drive and sexual function, which have their roots in biological and physiological processes. A medically based understanding of how these factors contribute to sex offending can result in both a better formulation of the cause of the problematic behaviour, and provide potentially powerful adjuncts to treatment (Figure 23.1).

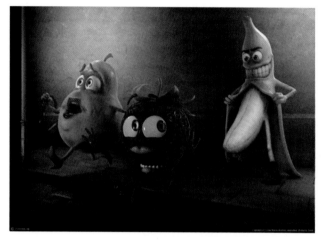

Figure 23.1 Sexual deviation. Source: http://alzhem.cgsociety.org/gallery/. Reproduced with permission from Jose Maria Andres Martin

Offending, deviance, disorder

When dealing with problematic sexual behaviour, a distinction needs to be made between behaviour that is illegal, behaviour that is deviant and behaviour that is associated with mental disorder, although there is often overlap between these categories (Box 23.1). In brief, sex offences are behaviours that are defined and proscribed by a society because of the harm they cause its citizens, sex deviance refers to behaviours that contravene the norms of society, while sexual disorders are conditions that are pathological in nature because they cause distress or dysfunction, and are formalized in diagnostic manuals such as the International Classification of Diseases (ICD) and the Diagnostic and Statistical Manual (DSM). When a behaviour moves into the realm of a disorder, doctors may become involved.

Box 23.1 **The distinction between offences, deviance and disorder**

- *Offences* defined by law. Vary over time and place. Can change quickly.
- *Deviance* determined by shared norms within a culture or subculture. A moral construct. Change is gradual.

ABC of Sexual Health, Third Edition. Edited by Kevan Wylie.
© 2015 John Wiley & Sons, Ltd. Published 2015 by John Wiley & Sons, Ltd.

- *Disorder* listed and defined in diagnostic manuals. Associated with dysfunction or distress. Change can be sudden with the introduction of a new edition of a diagnostic manual.

The manuals confuse matters, however, by identifying a specific type of sexual disorder – 'Disorders of Sexual Preference' in the ICD and 'Paraphilic Disorders' in the DSM – on the basis of both deviance and distress or dysfunction (although the ICD is less consistent in terms of the latter), and focusing on the description of behaviour rather than psychopathology (Box 23.2). The latest edition of the DSM (DSM-5) has muddied the waters even more by controversially labelling deviant sexual behaviour as a disorder if it involves a non-consenting person, even in cases where there is no distress or dysfunction in the person who displays it, further blurring the boundary between sex offence and sex disorder.

Thus, rape is an offence but may not be indicative of either deviance or a disorder, fetishism is sexually deviant but not an offence and often not a disorder, while sadism, which in many settings is not considered deviant but accepted as a 'minority interest', becomes both deviant and a disorder if it is problematic to an individual. Homosexuality used to satisfy all three categories, but in western societies now fits none.

Sexual behaviours such as hypersexuality or those associated with compulsive use of the internet to view pornography can cause marked distress or dysfunction in their own right, and can lead to offending. They are not recognized as mental disorders in the diagnostic manuals, but medical intervention may nonetheless be indicated.

Some individuals with mental illness may commit sex offences or engage in deviant sexual behaviour as a symptom of their illnesses rather than because of an underlying sexual disorder. For example, patients with hypomania may act in a sexually disinhibited manner,

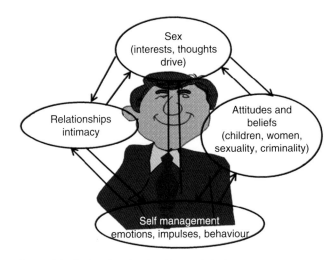

Figure 23.2 The four domains that drive sex behaviour

while psychotic individuals can act on delusions of a sexual nature. Substance misuse or brain disease may also unmask an otherwise well-controlled sexual pathology.

Assessment of sex offenders

Sex offending typically results from a combination of two or more of the domains shown in Figure 23.2. Although the psychologically minded doctor might take an interest in any of these areas, it is primarily the domain related to sex interests and drive, and to a lesser extent self-management, that medicine has most to offer.

We know little about what determines an individual's sexual arousal patterns, other than that they are not something about which he or she makes a conscious choice. Once sexual preferences are established, however, it is extremely difficult to change them. Where they result in illegal or dangerous behaviour if acted upon, the choice is to offend, to find alternative ways in which to satisfy sexual arousal, or to manage it better. Medical assessment and intervention is especially relevant to the last of these options.

The history should first obtain an account of the problem behaviour and associated fantasies and urges. Assessment then focuses on the characteristics of the sexual drive, the extent to which it is influenced by mood states, and the nature of the sexual fantasies (Box 23.3).

Box 23.2 **Key features of ICD and DSM definitions of disorders of sexual preference**

DSM-5

- recurrent
- persistent (lasting at least 6 months)
- intense
- involve deviant activity or target
- cause significant distress, impairment of functioning, or has acted on the sexual urge with a non-consenting person
- aged 18 or over

ICD-10
No specific unifying factors, but theme of:

- persistence
- strong preference
- deviant activity or target

Box 23.3 **The assessment of sexual drive**

Ask the patient
In the last 7 days:

- how many days did you masturbate to orgasm
- how many days did you masturbate not leading to orgasm
- on how many of those days did you masturbate more than once
- how many days did you engage in sexual behaviour with a partner
- on how many days did you engage in any type of sexual behaviour more than once

- in any one day, what is the maximum number of times you engaged in sexual activity

In general:

- do you think more about sex when you are feeling low or under stress
- are there other emotional states which affect how much you think about sex

In relation to the problematic sexual fantasies or behaviour

- about what percentage of your sexual thoughts relate to (the problematic fantasy or behaviour)

Have the patient rate the following in relation to the last 7 days:

Strength of sexual urges or fantasies

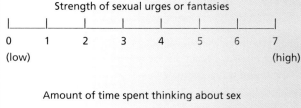

```
0    1    2    3    4    5    6    7
(low)                              (high)
```

Amount of time spent thinking about sex

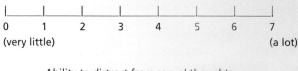

```
0    1    2    3    4    5    6    7
(very little)                      (a lot)
```

Ability to distract from sexual thoughts

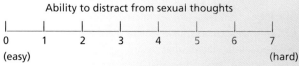

```
0    1    2    3    4    5    6    7
(easy)                             (hard)
```

Data from Kafka M P. Hypersexual desire in males: An operational definition and clinical implications for males with paraphilias and paraphilia-related disorders. *Archives of Sexual Behavior*, 1997, 26: 505–526.

The assessment aims to determine the degree of sexual preoccupation and rumination, the strength of the sex drive, and whether sex serves as a mood regulator. There is no agreed level of arousal that is diagnostic of high drive or excessive preoccupation. More useful is to obtain a general sense of the patient's sexual functioning and their subjective ability to manage it, and to establish a baseline for later treatment.

The biological basis of sexual arousal and targets for medical intervention

The neurobiological basis of sexual functioning is complex, and our knowledge of it is extremely limited. Testosterone receptors are found in many parts of the brain, while sexual arousal and behaviour are influenced by a range of neurotransmitters and hormones. Some exert their effects through general excitatory or inhibitory mechanisms, while others have a more specific impact. The most important neurotransmitters and hormones in terms of medical intervention are illustrated in Figure 23.3.

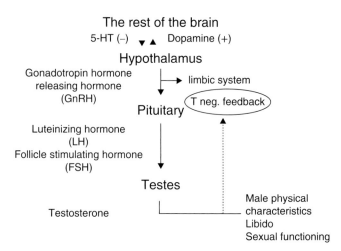

Figure 23.3 Important hormones in the control of sexual interest and functioning

Table 23.1 Drugs often used in sex offender treatment

Drug type	Examples
SSRIs	fluoxetine, sertraline
Mood stabilizers	lamotrigine, lithium
Dopamine antagonists	benperidol, other neuroleptics
Antiandrogens	cyproterone acetate
Progesterinics	medroxyprogesterone acetate
GnRH agonists	goserelin, leuprorelin, triptorelin

Drugs typically used in the treatment of sex offenders may interfere directly with the actions of testosterone, in which case they are referred to as anti-libidinals or antiandrogens, or they target neurotransmitter systems involved in sexual arousal and behaviour, especially serotonin and dopamine (Table 23.1).

Selective serotonin re-uptake inhibitors (SSRIs) have a general libido lowering effect. In addition, they can reduce the intensity and frequency of sexual fantasy and compulsive urges. They are of most benefit in patients with intrusive fantasies, or in whom problematic sexual behaviour is associated with strong urges, impulsivity or low mood. Although potentially of value in any type of offending, they should especially be considered in exhibitionists and internet downloaders. Dose levels used in obsessive–compulsive disorder are typically required.

Mood stabilizers may be of benefit where sexual fantasy or behaviour appears to act as a mood regulator, with variability in mood associated with changes in the frequency of sexual fantasy or behaviour.

The reduction in sexual arousal caused by dopamine antagonists is probably caused by an increase in prolactin levels (dopamine inhibits prolactin release). The effect on arousal, however, is variable and unreliable.

The antiandrogens, progesterinics and GnRH agonists all work by inhibiting the activity of testosterone in one way or another. They have a powerful libido lowering effect, which is seen as a loss of sexual interest. They also impair sexual functioning. They are most appropriate, and can be of great benefit, in individuals who have

Table 23.2 The use of testosterone-lowering drugs

Drug	Typical Dose	Comments
cyproterone acetate	50–200 mg/day oral	Not available in USA Depot available in some countries
medroxyprog-esterone acetate	300–500 mg/wk im 50–100 mg/day oral	Rarely used in Europe
goserelin	3.6 mg/month or 10.8 mg/3 monthly im	A testosterone receptor blocker is used in the first weeks when prescribed for prostate cancer, but this is probably not necessary when used as an antilibidinal.
leuprorelin	3.75–7.5 mg/month or 11.25 mg/3 monthly im	
triptorelin	3.75 mg/month or 11.25 mg/3 monthly im	

None of these drugs should be used in persons under 18 years of age because of effects on bone maturation.

Table 23.3 Monitoring the use of testosterone-lowering drugs

	Initial visit	3 months	6 months	Annual[a]
Full blood count	X			X
Liver function	X	X	X	X
Glucose	X	X	X	X
Renal function	X	X	X	X
Thyroid	X			X
Lipids (not fasting)	X	X	X	X
Testosterone	X	X	If indicated	X
Cortisol	If indicated			If indicated
Bone density	X (GnRH agonist)			X (GnRH agonist[b])
Weight	X			X
Physical examination (esp. cvs, breast)	X			X

[a]After 1 year, investigations are carried out annually unless otherwise indicated.
[b]Typically every 3 years, but may be more frequent in older men.

high levels of sex drive and arousal. Their potent side-effect profile, however, means that their use needs to be closely monitored, with regular physical examination and investigations (Tables 23.2 and 23.3, Box 23.4). Patients should be advised to make lifestyle changes to improve their cardiovascular and bone health (i.e. weight loss, increased exercise, stop smoking and similar steps).

Box 23.4 **Most common side effects of testosterone-lowering drugs**

- weight gain
- hot flushes
- fatigue
- muscle weakness
- depression
- gynaecomastia
- endocrine abnormalities
- liver function abnormalities (cyproterone acetate)
- hypertension, thromboembolism
- bone demineralization
- impotence
- infertility

Table 23.4 Treatment algorithm based on presentation (plus psychological treatment in most cases)

Presentation	Treatment
High levels of sexual rumination or preoccupation	SSRI in OCD doses; if unsuccessful then oral antiandrogen
Fantasy or behaviour associated with mood dysregulation	If depression, SSRI; if variability in mood, mood stabilizer
Compulsive or impulsive aspect to sexual behaviour	SSRI in OCD doses; if unsuccessful then oral antiandrogen
High sex drive	Oral antiandrogen, if unsuccessful then GnRH agonist

Treatment algorithms

The World Federation of Societies of Biological Psychiatry (WFSBP) has produced guidelines for 'the biological treatment of paraphilias'. Its algorithm is based primarily on risk, with increasing levels of risk associated with more potent medication that has greater impact on sexual activity and desire. Although sensible, this type of approach could result in prescribing for reasons of social control rather than for medical indications.

An alternative is to base treatment on the phenomenological presentation, with risk a secondary consideration (Table 23.4). In this case, the doctor does not assume primary responsibility for public safety, but contributes to it by assisting the offender address those factors which make him more likely to reoffend. Risk is left to be managed by individuals working in the criminal justice system. Conversely, there is no reason why a 'low risk' offender should not be prescribed an antiandrogen if the level of his drive justifies it.

In either case, so long as the offender has capacity then medication to suppress sexual arousal should only be prescribed with consent, the patient having been informed of the medications' risks and benefits, particularly given the potential harm that can be caused by testosterone-lowering drugs.

Consideration also needs to be given to confidentiality. Unless the offender-patient discloses information which suggests someone is at risk, he is entitled to the same levels of confidentiality as any other patient. Good practice, however, is to share information with others involved in his management with his consent.

Further reading

American Psychiatric Association (2013) *Paraphilic Disorders in Diagnostic and Statistical Manual of Mental Disorders, (DSM-5)*, 5th edn. American Psychiatric Association, Arlington, VA.

Bancroft, J. & Vukadinovic, Z. (2004) Sexual addiction, sexual compulsivity, sexual impulse disorder or what? Towards a theoretical model. *Journal of Sex Research*, **41**, 225–234.

Grubin, D. (2008) Medical models and interventions in sexual deviance. In: Laws, D.R. & O'Donohue, W. (eds), *Sexual Deviance: Theory, Assessment and Treatment*, 2nd edn. The Guilford Press, New York.

Grubin, D., Middleton, D., Craissati, J. & Gordon, H. (2014) Disordered and offensive sexual behavior. In: Gunn, J. & Taylor, P.J. (eds), *Forensic Psychia-try: Clinical, Legal and Ethical Issues*, 2nd edn. Taylor & Francis Group, Boca Raton, FL.

Rosler, A. & Witztum, E. (2000) Pharmacotherapy of paraphilias in the next millennium. *Behavioral Sciences and the Law*, **18**, 43–56.

Thibaut, F., De La Barra, F., Gordon, H., Cosysns, P. & Bradford, J.M.W. (2010) The World Federation of Societies of Biological Psychiatry (WFSBP) Guidelines for the biological treatment of paraphilias. *World Journal of Biological Psychiatry*, **11**, 604–655.

CHAPTER 24

Ethnic and Cultural Aspects of Sexuality

Sara Nasserzadeh

Psychosexual Therapist, Connections ABC, New York, NY, USA

OVERVIEW

- Multicultural and multiethnic societies such as the UK warrant a healthcare workforce that is competent in working with diversity

- Sexual health issues have a strong cultural and ethnic dimension, which impacts their epidemiology, assessment and treatment strategies

- Male and female sexual behaviours, genital surgeries and modifications, vaginal practices, hymen dilemmas, rapid ejaculation, dyspareunia and vaginismus are influenced by cultural and ethnic backgrounds of patients

- In history taking, sexual terminology of a patient from a different cultural or ethnic background might be different, which may influence the direction and outcome of the consultation

- Once the health care professional (HCP) suspects or establishes the cultural determinants of a sexual health condition, help in the form of consultation with an experienced cross-cultural counsellor or therapist may be appropriate.

Introduction

Religious and cultural beliefs are known to have great influence on individuals' health belief and behaviour. These beliefs not only influence how healthy sexual behaviour is defined, but also it has a significant impact on the patient–HCP alliance and the treatment process, which ultimately influences the outcomes.

Based on 2011 census in the UK, 19.5% of the England and Wales population are not categorized as White British (almost 1 in 5). The majority of other ethnicities in the UK consist of people with ethnic or cultural backgrounds from South Asia (particularly from India and Pakistan), Africa, Caribbean region, other parts of Asia, Middle East and Europe as well as people with mixed ethnicities. After the 'White British' category, Indian was the next largest ethnic group with 1.4 million people (2.5%) followed by Pakistani (2.0%). The remaining ethnic groups each accounted for up to 2% of the population in 2011.

Just a glance at medical textbooks and literature written for HCPs can provide a sense that most of these materials have been written to address the white populations. It might have made sense statistically, because they represented the majority of the UK population; however, the demographics are changing and there are certain conditions and presenting problems that are more often presented by the minority groups. In addition, there are subtle considerations to the common complaints by all groups that could be misunderstood or mismanaged for the minority groups if the practitioner looks at the issue through the lens he or she uses to address the White British patients. To bridge this cultural knowledge gap, some HCPs would refer those cases to colleagues who might be more familiar with that specific culture; however, this might not be feasible especially if he/she is the only local HCP or the patient would not feel comfortable to see a person from his or her community for sexual issues.

These perspectives could range from viewing one's sexuality as private matter to the extreme of believing that one's sexuality may influence the wellbeing of cosmos and the fertility of earth. From a moral values perspective, some people may regard sexuality as a positive force to be celebrated and some may view it as an ultimate sin and a source of all evils. To make the context even more complex, there is a striking difference even amongst the same ethnic group who might check the same ethnicity box in their registration forms. By reading through these lines, the practitioner may realize how these beliefs could influence the patient's perspective and their behaviour towards their sexuality, the way in which they talk about it and the importance and emphasis one might put on it.

In this chapter, we will review some topics that have a cultural or ethnic dimension to them and knowing that background could assist in the diagnosis and treatment process.

Genital surgeries and modifications

Male circumcision is perhaps one of the oldest genital modification surgeries practiced around the world. Although it is mostly common and required in male newborns with Moslem or Jewish backgrounds, certain Christian-dominant countries such as the United States also practice it commonly. Male circumcision is not required or practiced in Hinduism or Buddhism. Circumcised men typically have no complaints rather than occasional questions regarding the linkage of foreskin or the lack of it with one's sexual satisfaction and its potential contribution to oversensitivity and rapid ejaculation.

ABC of Sexual Health, Third Edition. Edited by Kevan Wylie.

For women, the term circumcision is sometimes wrongly used to represent various degrees of genital cutting.[1] Genital cutting is a cultural practice, which can be performed at different stages of life such as before puberty, before one's wedding or right after the birth of the first child. Asking about any previous genital surgeries or modifications can assist the HCPs in assessing conditions such as pain disorders, bleeding after sex and in recurring cases of bacterial vaginosis and genital herpes infections, which are reported to be more common amongst women who had various degrees of genital modifications. This practice is more common in certain African countries, some parts of Southeast Asia (such as Malaysia) and parts of the Middle East. Although this condition is referred to as genital mutilation in ICD-10-CM (code: N90.81), the use of this term in a consultation with a patient can be patronizing and therefore not recommended. Many women perceive this procedure as a form of cosmetic beautification, moral enhancement or dignifying improvement of the appearance of the human body. Some who are not satisfied with the outcome of these procedures or suffer from its complications may request referrals for reconstructive surgeries and modifications.

Vaginal and penile practices

Some cultures and ethnicities have specific penile and vaginal practices[2] that may predispose patients to certain health conditions or interfere with contraceptive recommendations or medical treatments. Excessive vaginal douching (seen, e.g. within the US amongst particular groups such as African-Americans), which is strongly influenced by one's sociocultural beliefs and perception of cleanliness, has been shown to predispose women to a variety of health conditions including bacterial vaginosis. In certain cultures (e.g. in Mozambique and South Africa), it might be women who may insist on not using condoms due to a desire to have skin-to-skin friction and a belief that semen can have health benefits for them. It is also well established that cultural beliefs may negatively influence adherence to vaginal medical treatments, especially if the women is asked to apply the medication topically or inside the vagina. As a result of that, it is critical for an HCP to ask specific questions about vaginal practices (in a broad sense) and ensure there are no reservations to adherence due to cultural and ethnic belief systems.

Within each culture there might be varieties that could be missed by a physician who is not familiar with the genital practices within that culture (even from someone from that culture). This will add to the importance of a comprehensive history taking. For example, there are reports of casual penile practices (intentional fracturing of the penis to hear who makes a louder noise) within a small

[1] The term Genital Cutting is used intentionally in this chapter instead of the widely used Genital Mutilation, which could be a patronizing term that does not resonate with the women who have undergone the procedure. The Female Genital Mutilation Act 2003 prevents British citizens and permanent residents from assisting or carrying out FGM in the UK or abroad.

[2] The term vaginal practices is broadly defined to include all efforts to wash, modify, cut, cleanse, enhance, dry, tighten, lubricate or loosen the vagina, labia, clitoris or hymen. This could include a substance or material applied, ingested, inserted or steamed.

population in Iran. These patients' main complaints are usually either difficulty with erection or an asymmetrical penis.

Hymen dilemmas

The hymen is considered in some cultures especially in the Middle East and North African countries as a proof that the woman is still a virgin, pure and untouched. Therefore, young women who had pre-marital sex but are from such backgrounds may seek hymenoplasty or request a medical certificate confirming that the hymen in intact. The HCP might face women seeking this treatment, and many feel the need for a guideline for such cases, as they had to use their own judgement for referral to a plastic surgeon, social services or gynae-cologists not knowing which would be more effective. In almost all cases, counselling on the existing myths and educating the women seeking this treatment has been proven effective. On another front, because this procedure may have been offered in other countries or at illegal or private settings, the HCPs may encounter complications of this procedure in the form of infections, bleeding and pain.

Rapid ejaculation

Rapid ejaculation is one of the main reasons that men seek help from urologists, general practitioners and psychosexual therapists worldwide; however, research shows that the presentation of this problem to the clinics are significantly higher in certain ethnicities. Some studies have concluded that this problem is more common in men from Muslim and Asian backgrounds. As there are cultural and religious factors involved in this problem, a consultation with or referral to a psychosexual therapist might be beneficial in addition to standard medical therapies.

Dyspareunia and vaginismus

The presentation of dyspareunia and vaginismus in the context of culture and ethnicity has been reported to be higher amongst certain groups such as Muslims, Hindus and Jewish people. This might be due to negative attitudes towards sex, value attached to one's virginity, misinformation regarding the first sexual encounter, lack of education and sexual techniques in both partners and sometimes a sudden change of status from single and virgin to married and sexually open. In addition to pain, these couples may seek help for infertility or unconsummated marriages. Once the organic causes are ruled out, sex education plus a consultation with a qualified psychosexual therapist is advisable.

Heterosexual men having casual sex with men (masculine socialization)

In certain cultures (or subcultures), heterosexual men could have casual sex with other men, which may create a confusing picture for an HCP. When asking the questions, they may not see this information relevant and therefore not disclose it, as they mostly do not regard themselves as 'bisexual' or 'homosexual', even may be offended by these terminologies. However, if the questions are asked without a reference to any labels or categories, patients may disclose information that they would not have otherwise. This could

Box 24.1 **How to adjust a consultation based on culture and ethnicity of the patient**

Use of an interpreter	If possible, use an independent interpreter of the same gender as the patient and not a family member
Privacy	Asking more sensitive questions in a questionnaire to be filled before the session and then use their answers as prompts to bring the matter up (e.g. erectile dysfunction (ED) in diabetic patients)
Gender of the HCP	If the primary presenting problem is a sexual issue, it might be helpful to offer a consultation with an HCP who has the same gender
Ethnic background of the HCP	While having the same background might help at occasions, but in small communities patients may prefer seeing someone from outside of that community
Lexicon	Choice of word and the way a person explains his or her issues might be different from how it is discussed by the HCP.

- 'Weakness' could be a description of ED. Or 'back pain' could be an indirect way of discussing his concerns with masturbation.
- The definition of terms such as 'cleanliness', 'dry sex' needs to be discussed on an individual basis.
- In certain cultures, 'sex' only refers to 'penile–vaginal intercourse'. Oral and anal sex is not considered sex.

be quite important in the context of assessing sexually transmitted infections (STIs) and HIV infection.

History taking in multiethnic multicultural context

There are certain elements of history taking that may need to be adjusted based on a cultural or ethnic background of the patient. A summary of those points is listed in Box 24.1.

Conclusion

Some presenting problems are more common in patients from certain cultures or ethnicities. But in most cases, it is fairly consistent across the board. However, what is significantly different is the context of the same problem and its underlying factors. This can influence how the problem is communicated to the HCP, which then can impact the assessment and treatment plans. This chapter was a brief introduction to the importance of cultural context and the nuances that HCPs need to be aware of.

Further reading

Diclemente, R.J., Young, A.M., Painter, J.L., Wingood, G.M., Rose, E. & Sales, J.M. (2012) Prevalence and correlates of recent vaginal douching among African American adolescent females. *Journal of Pediatric and Adolescent Gynecology*, **25** (**1**), 48–53.

Essén, B., Blomkvist, A., Helström, L. & Johnsdotter, S. (2010) The experience and responses of Swedish health professionals to patients requesting virginity restoration (hymen repair). *Reproductive Health Matters*, **18** (**35**), 38–46.

Eşsizoğlu, A., Yasan, A., Yildirim, E.A., Gurgen, F. & Ozkan, M. (2011) Double standard for traditional value of virginity and premarital sexuality in Turkey: a university students case. *Women and Health*, **51** (**2**), 136–150.

Frewen, A., Rapee, R.M., Bowden, P. & Lagios, K. (2007) Regional differences in men attending a sexual health clinic in Sydney for premature ejaculation. *Journal of Sexual Medicine*, **4** (**6**), 1733–1738.

Hall, K.S. & Graham, C.A. (eds) (2013) *The Cultural Context of Sexual Pleasure and Problems: Psychotherapy with Diverse Clients*. Routledge, England.

Khodary, M.M., Shazly, S.A., Ali, M.K., Badee, A.Y. & Shaaban, O.M. (2013) The patterns and criteria of vaginal douching and the risk of preterm labor among upper Egypt women. *Journal of Lower Genital Tract Disease*, **17** (**4**), e35.. doi:10.1097/LGT.0b013e3182a4e7a5.

Luong, M.L., Libman, M., Dahhou, M. *et al.* (2010) Vaginal douching, bacterial vaginosis, and spontaneous preterm birth. *Journal of Obstetrics and Gynaecology Canada*, **32** (**4**), 313–320.

Malebranche, D., Fields, E., Bryant, L. & Harper, S. (2009) Masculine socialization and sexual risk behaviors among black men who have sex with men: a qualitative exploration. *Men and Masculinities*, **12** (**1**), 90–112.

Martin Hilber, A., Hull, T.H., Preston-Whyte, E. *et al.* (2010) A cross-cultural study of vaginal practices and sexuality: implications for sexual health. *Social Science and Medicine*, **70** (**3**), 392–400.

van Moorst, B.R., van Lunsen, R.H., van Dijken, D.K. & Salvatore, C.M. (2012) Backgrounds of women applying for hymen reconstruction, the effects of counselling on myths and misunderstandings about virginity, and the results of hymen reconstruction. *European Journal of Contraception & Reproductive Health Care*, **17** (**2**), 93–105.

Office for National Statistics (2011) Part of 2011 Census, Key Statistics for Local Authorities in England and Wales Release. Ethnicity and National Identity in England and Wales 2011, Published in December 2011.

Richardson, D. & Goldmeier, D. (2005) Premature ejaculation--does country of origin tell us anything about etiology? *Journal of Sexual Medicine*, **2** (**4**), 508–512.

Zargooshi, J. (2004) Trauma as the cause of Peyronie's disease: penile fracture as a model of trauma. *Journal of Urology*, **172** (**1**), 186–188.

Zargooshi, J. (2009) Sexual function and tunica albuginea wound healing following penile fracture: an 18-year follow-up study of 352 patients from Kermanshah, Iran. *Journal of Sexual Medicine*, **6** (**4**), 1141–1150.

CHAPTER 25

Concerns Arising from Sexual Orientation, Practices and Behaviours

Dominic Davies

Pink Therapy, London, UK

> **OVERVIEW**
>
> This chapter will explore patients' worries
> - about being gay/lesbian or attractions to the same-sex.
> - about amount of sex they are having or the circumstances surrounding it.
> - about sexual fantasies or sexual behaviours which they feel are outside the 'norm' including bondage and discipline, dominance and submission, sadism and masochism (BDSM)/Kink.

Discussing sexuality issues with health care professionals is often fraught with anxiety on the part of the patient for fear of being judged and also on the part of the professional because of embarrassment, lack of training and personal moral values and beliefs of the professional, which might conflict with, or impede, open and accepting patient-centred health care. It is crucial to be comfortable with discussing sexuality issues and to remember that you are their doctor, not their spiritual advisor or moral guardian.

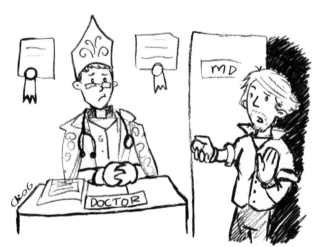

"OH SORRY, I THINK I HAVE THE WRONG ROOM..."

Source: © Chris Gould 2014 http://www.cgsketchbook.com/. Reproduced with permission.

ABC of Sexual Health, Third Edition. Edited by Kevan Wylie.
© 2015 John Wiley & Sons, Ltd. Published 2015 by John Wiley & Sons, Ltd.

Worries about same-sex sexual attractions

The British government when estimating the possible take up of Civil Partnerships estimated around 5–7% of the population are lesbian or gay. Whilst it is very difficult to conduct accurate research into sexual behaviour, UK government statisticians have generated these estimates based on best evidence. A greater number of people engage in same-sex sexual behaviour from time to time but may not identify as lesbian gay or bisexual. For the vast majority of these, their same-sex attractions will not cause them any difficulties or concerns.

Homosexuality was declassified as a mental illness by the WHO in 1991 and it is now accepted by all leading medical and psychological bodies that homosexuality and bisexuality (now referred to as being lesbian, gay or bisexual) is perfectly normal. Due to religious, ethnic and cultural beliefs there will still be some people who present for help in changing their sexual orientation. There is no reputable evidence that sexual re-orientation therapies are effective: indeed, a fair amount has accrued showing that such methods can be, at best, harmful and, at worst, result in serious self-harm, depression and even suicide.

Responding to the unhappy homosexual

Clinicians faced with requests for change need to explain the above sensitively and refer the patient for psychological support in finding ways to integrate their sexuality with other areas of their lives. It may not be advisable or safe for everyone to 'come out' (openly declare their sexual orientation) and so encouraging the patient to find a good balance between those who know and accept them fully and those who do not know can be one of the tasks of therapeutic intervention.

From time to time someone will present to you who is deeply concerned and conflicted about their same-sex attractions. This person is likely to be male and may come from a faith background which forbids homosexuality. If your own cultural background or religious beliefs also suggest that homosexuality is somehow inherently 'against nature' or 'God's Will' then you might be inclined to agree to their request for help to change their orientation. This is likely to feel even more acutely relevant if the person is suicidal or facing family and community rejection if they were to come out.

It is important to make clear that there is absolutely no evidence to show that *any* psychological or physical treatment exists to cure homosexuality. As it is not a disease, this may be obvious, but homosexuality often becomes caught up in spiritual, religious and cultural debates which may make it difficult to retain the medical and ethical principles of the Hippocratic Oath and *do no harm*. Even colluding with the idea that cure might be possible, or a reduction in same-sex desire achievable, you are reinforcing the notion that homosexuality is wrong. Failed attempts to resolve this issue by so-called '*reparative therapies*' are likely to result in suicidal depression.

The most appropriate treatment option is referral to a knowledgeable and non-judgemental counsellor or psychologist either through a local lesbian, gay, bisexual and transgender (LGBT) helpline or via the online Directory of Pink Therapists (www.pinktherapy.com).

Mental health concerns

It should be born in mind that many lesbian, gay and bisexual people experience higher incidence of anxiety, depression and self-harm and alcohol and substance misuse due to living in a society which stigmatizes them and this is not due to their same-sex attractions per se. Recent research has shown that bisexual people have poorer mental health than lesbian women and gay men. This is likely to be due to prejudice against bisexual people (biphobia) within both heterosexual and lesbian and gay, communities.

Pharmacotherapy for depression

Physicians might want to consider the sexual side-effects of selective serotonin re-uptake inhibitor (SSRI)-based medications when treating gay and bisexual men for depression as these frequently cause a loss of libido, erectile dysfunction or ejaculatory difficulties and this can both compound the depression and low self-worth further, and have implications which affect adherence and treatment compliance. Not all SSRIs have these effects but it maybe useful to consider this aspect before pharmacotherapy begins.

Recreational drug use

It can also be helpful – especially in major cities with large gay male communities – to explore recreational drug use and refer patients to specialist agencies for help where appropriate. Increasing sexualized use of certain recreational drugs, such as gamma-hydroxybutyric acid (GHB), gamma-butyrolactone (GBL), Methamphetamine (Crystal Meth/Tina) and Mephedrone (MCAT/Miaow-Miaow), have been implicated in increased HIV and hepatitis C infections – amongst other sexually transmitted infections (STIs) – as well as affecting compliance with antiretroviral therapy in HIV+ve gay men.

Consensual non-monogamies

There are several forms of consensual non-monogamy and not everyone buys into the idea that they can only have sex and love with one person for life (mononormativity). In some cultures,

polygamy is supported and in the West we see various forms of consensual non-monogamy. For example 50–80% of gay men tend to be in open relationships after 5 years or so. Many heterosexual couples enjoy partner sharing/swapping and might privately engage in 'swinging' to spice up their sexual relationship. Others recognize that they can love more than one person and would identify as polyamorous and maintain open and committed relationships with more than one partner. Avoid assuming that the mention of one sexual/romantic partner means there would not be any other ones or that non-monogamy itself is problematic or pathological.

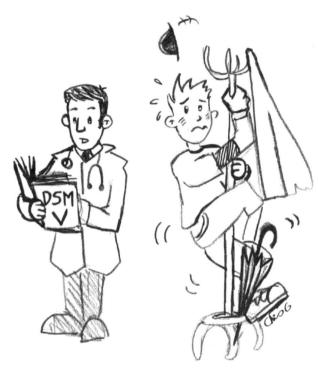

"WELL, AS SEXUAL ADDICTION DOESN'T EXIST, I THINK IT MUST BE RESTLESS GROIN SYNDROME..."

Source: © Chris Gould 2014 http://www.cgsketchbook.com/. Reproduced with permission.

Concerns about sexual activity

Some patients (generally men of all sexual orientations) may present with concerns about the amount of sex they are having or the circumstances in which they are having it. These concerns might be their own or motivated by concerns from their partners/family members. They may believe they suffer from 'Sexual Addiction'. This populist diagnosis is highly contested and was recently reviewed by the psychiatric nomenclature committee of the American Psychiatric Association, who decided against including *Hypersexual Desire Disorder* in the latest revision of diagnostic and statistical manual of mental disorder (DSM) V. 'Sexual Addiction' is a controversial pseudo-diagnosis with highly variable and clinically unreliable diagnostic criteria.

This is not to say that sexually compulsive behaviour does not exist or that sexual desire and sexual behaviour might well get out

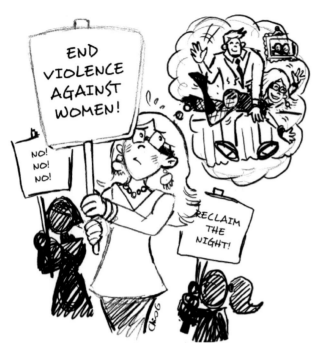

"WE GET TURNED ON AT NIGHT BY THE VERY SAME THINGS
THAT WE WILL DEMONSTRATE AGAINST DURING THE DAY."
(PEREL, 2013)

Source: © Chris Gould 2014 http://www.cgsketchbook.com/. Reproduced
with permission.

of control at various points in someone's life – due to either stress
or anxiety or as an aspect of deeper psychopathology in the form of
a personality disorder or depressive illness, which may predispose
someone to compulsive sexual acting out or risk taking. A careful
assessment of the whole person, not one which focuses solely
on their sexual behaviour, however lurid, bizarre and intriguing
that might be, is essential for a holistic approach to sexual and
mental health.

There is some evidence that some people have higher than average levels of testosterone (High T) so that a higher sex drive is normal and healthy for them. It is not uncommon for people who have
High T to be able to engage in sex four or five times a day and
become stressed and anxious if they are unable to orgasm. It can
be problematic and distressing when someone with High T is in a
relationship with someone who has a lower (or perhaps suppressed)
sexual drive. A referral to a specialist sex and relationship therapist
to explore these issues can frequently be helpful.

The underlying principle to keep in mind in working with anyone
on sexual issues is whether the activity is causing physical or psychological damage to themselves or another person. We might also
want to consider whether the patient or their partner(s) are feeling
coerced into sex or alternative sexual behaviours. If the behaviour
is non-coercive and involves no long-term damage then it is more
helpful for the clinician to simply reassure the patient about trans-
gressive or alternative sexual practices, and to help them manage
feelings of guilt or shame about them.

Sexual expression and desire can be tied into a deep well of guilt,
shame and misinformation that leads many people to feel bad about

their sexual behaviour or fantasies and acceptance and reassurance
from a trusted professional can do much to alleviate this guilt and
anxiety. There has been major research into sexual fantasies which
demonstrates a wide range of erotic imaginings which are often dis-
cordant with the individual's own values, beliefs and moral code.

BDSM/kink – assessing risk

BDSM (also known as Kink) are sexual practices which involve an
explicit and consensual use of power exchange and sometimes sensation to control or increase erotic and sexual pleasure.

These practices involve people of all sexual orientations and
genders. Those outside the BDSM/Kink community are often
concerned about the physical and mental well-being of those who
engage in these activities and potential risks, believing they will
always involve pain and are dangerous.

When considering risk, it can be helpful to know whether the person engaged in kink is doing so under one of two common codes of
behaviour – Safe, Sane and Consensual (SSC) or Risk Aware Consensual Kink (RACK). RACK came about as an acknowledgment
that some activities (e.g. breath control, engaging in blood play and
surface piercings) involve some risks to health and that the people
involved are aware of these dangers and well informed of the risks.
It can also be helpful to check out whether the person is involved to
some extent in a Kink community (either online or in the real world)
and has social support from peers for their sexual activities, as this
ensures a kind of safety net, mentoring and sources of information
and support.

Psycho-education

Some people may be concerned about their sexual desires or
behaviours and may benefit from some psycho-educational support. Websites like Fetlife (www.fetlife.com) demonstrate an enor-
mous range of fetishes and activities and their forums are replete
with supportive advice and information to which patients can be
usefully directed. There are also several guides to BDSM activities
and the psychology of BDSM (see especially works by Dossie
Easton, a San Francisco-based psychotherapist and sex therapist).

There is a commonly held myth that BDSM is inherently pathological and likely to be a result of early abuse. Various research studies have shown this to be false and that BDSM should be considered
a recreational activity and a good argument has also been made for
it being thought of as a sexual orientation.

Further reading

Anton, B.S. (2010) Proceedings of the American Psychological Association for the legislative year 2009: Minutes of the annual meeting of the
Council of Representatives and minutes of the meetings of the Board
of Directors. *American Psychologist*, **65**, 385–475.. doi:10.1037/a0019553
online http://www.apa.org/about/policy/sexual-orientation.aspx Accessed
4/12/2013.

Barker, M., Richards, C., Jones, R., Bowes-Catton, H., Plowman, T., Yockney,
J. & Morgan, M. (2012) The Bisexuality Report. Available for download
http://www.open.ac.uk/ccig/files/ccig/The%20BisexualityReport%20Feb.
2012.pdf Accessed 4/12/2014.

Connolly, P.H., Haley, H., Gendelman, J. & Miller, J. (2006) Psychological functioning of bondage/domination/sado-masochism practitioners. *Journal of Psychology & Human Sexuality*, **18**, 79–120.

Fearless Press (2013) Is BDSM a Matter of Sexual Orientation. Online blog: http://www.fearlesspress.com/2013/03/17/is-bdsm-a-matter-of-sexual-orientation/ Accessed 27/05/2013.

Khar, B. (2007) *Sex and the Psyche: The Truth About Our Most Secret Fantasies.* Penguin, London.

Ley, D. (2012) *The Myth of Sex Addiction.* Rowman & Littlefield Publishers, Plymouth.

Newmahr, S. (2010) Rethinking kink: sadomasochism as serious leisure. *Qualitative Sociology*, **33**, 313–331.

Ortmann, D. & Sprott, R. (2013) *Sexual Outsiders: Understanding BDSM Sexualities and Communities.* Rowman & Littlefield Publishers, Plymouth.

Perel, E. (2013) The Secret to Desire in a Long-Term Relationship. http://www.ted.com/talks/esther_perel_the_secret_to_desire_in_a_long_term_relationship.html Accessed 27/05/2013.

Richards, C. & Barker, M. (2013) *Sexuality & Gender for Counsellors, Psychologists and Other Health Professionals: a practical guide.* Sage, London.

Richters, J., De Visser, R.O., Rissel, C.E., Grulich, A.E. & Smith, A.M.A. (2008) Demographic and psychosocial features of participants in bondage and discipline, "Sadomasochism" or dominance and submission (BDSM): data from a national survey. *Journal of Sexual Medicine*, **5**, 1660–1688.

Stuart, D. (2013) Sexualised drug use by MSM: background, current status and response. *HIV Nursing Journal*, **13** (**1**), 6–10 (Spring 2013).

Wismeijer, A.A.J. & van Assen, M.A.L.M. (2013) Psychological characteristics of BDSM practitioners. *Journal of Sexual Medicine*, **10** (**8**), 1943–1952.

CHAPTER 26

Gender Dysphoria and Transgender Health

Lin Fraser[1] and Gail A. Knudson[2]

[1]San Francisco, CA, USA
[2]University of British Columbia, Vancouver BC, Canada

OVERVIEW

- The field is evolving towards health care and away from pathology
- Term 'gender dysphoria' strives to seek a balance to depathologize yet still allow access to care
- Our understanding of the condition has changed and it is no longer seen as a disorder. No one's identity is a disorder; the diagnosis is based on the distress of mind/body incongruence
- The World Professional Association of Transgender Health (WPATH) publish health care guidelines (Standards of Care (SOC)) which have changed over time to reflect changes in how the condition is understood
- Treatment is individualized and medical care is based on symtomatology and the degree of relief of dysphoria
- Interventions may include feminizing and masculinizing hormone therapy and gender affirming surgery depending on the needs of the individual
- Transgender individuals have a high rate of mental health concerns.

Introduction

What is in a name?

Language matters when discussing transgender health. The field is evolving towards health, away from pathology, with language following suit. The word transgender is generally seen as an umbrella term that covers the spectrum of transsexual, transgender and gender nonconforming identities. Gender dysphoria is the medical term describing the distress that emerges from body/mind incongruence.

Language and terminology are continually moving in the field and terms used in this chapter will likely change even before publication. Different terms may describe parallel experiences and may arise from different cultural understandings. Some names are more likely to be used by transgender people themselves out of an increasingly vocal and proud trans community.

Physician Dr. Norman Fisk coined the name 'gender dysphoria' in 1979 during the early years of the new field. Dysphoria is derived

from the Greek word *dysphoros* meaning 'hard to bear'. Fisk used the term gender dysphoria, to describe the situation he was seeing in his patients where the gender they had been assigned at birth, based on their natal sex, was hard to bear. They sought treatment to alleviate this dysphoria.

Over the years, terms used in the medical nomenclature to describe this condition have included gender dysphoria, transsexualism and gender identity disorder. Usage of the term, gender dysphoria, strives to seek a balance to depathologize yet still allow access to health care. Professional consensus is that no one's identity is a disorder; the diagnosis is based on the distress caused by the gender dysphoria.

Transgender beyond disorder and evolution of the standards of care – how did we get here?

Trans people have existed in all cultures and across time. Conditions similar to the Western conception of gender dysphoria appear across cultures and throughout known history. Some famous people are said to have had discomfort with their anatomical or assigned sex, including the Roman Emperor Heliogabalus, James I of England, and Henry III of France. As long ago as Hippocrates' times in the fifth century BC, male to female changes were reported in a Caucasian tribe. Similar groups in ancient Tahitian tribes and North American Aboriginals were described as having special spiritual powers.

Evolution of medical treatment

Magnus Hirschfeld introduced the term transsexual in 1923. In 1930, the first sexual reassignment surgery was performed. In 1954, Harry Benjamin was the first physician to distinguish transsexualism from same-sex attraction. He described a case series of non-psychotic men who self-castrated to relieve distress.

The Harry Benjamin International Gender Dysphoria Association, HBIGDA (now the WPATH (The World Professional Association for Transgender Health)), an interdisciplinary group of mental health professionals, endocrinologists, surgeons, and other professionals treating gender dysphoria, was formed in 1977. This collaboration led to the development of ethical standardized treatment guidelines, SOC, by the newly formed organization. The first SOC were published in 1979 (and the latest, SOC7, were published in 2011).

ABC of Sexual Health, Third Edition. Edited by Kevan Wylie.
© 2015 John Wiley & Sons, Ltd. Published 2015 by John Wiley & Sons, Ltd.

The first Standards were developed to improve the field and to protect trans people from unscrupulous surgeons who were operating 'on demand' which resulted in many unfortunate outcomes. The SOC have changed over time to reflect changes in how the condition is understood. Country-specific (e.g. UK) SOC have been influenced by the successive WPATH guidelines.

Diagnostic codes in the DSM and ICD

Transsexualism was first included in the American Psychiatric Association's Diagnostic and Statistical Manual of Mental Disorders, third revision (DSM III) (1980) and DSM III-R (1987). The term was replaced by Gender Identity Disorder in DSM IV (1994) and DSM-IV-TR (2000). DSM-5 uses the original term, coined by Fisk, Gender Dysphoria.

The World Health Organization's International Classification of Diseases (ICDs) has followed suit. In ICD-9, the condition transsexualism was classified under 'Sexual deviation and disorders', in ICD-10 as Gender Identity Disorder, under Sexual and Gender Identity Disorders. The team responsible for the nomenclature in ICD-11, due to be published in 2017 will use depathologizing language yet to be determined.

Gender is a matter of identity not disorder

When the first SOC and diagnoses were written, the assumption was that trans people seeking treatment would move from one sex to another, requiring cross-sex hormones and sex-reassignment surgery to alleviate the gender dysphoria. The paradigm was based on a gender binary and an opposite-sex model.

Gender is now seen as a spectrum, rather than a binary, with many variations along the way and health care is more individualized. The change over time is in response to new knowledge and the rise of trans community in the 1990s. More trans providers are lending their voices to their own health care. Gender is a matter of identity not disorder.

Now, we are moving away from classifying transgender identities as a disorder and seeing them as normal variations on a gender spectrum. Some see transgender rights as the civil rights issue of our time because of the stigma and marginalization that still exists.

Our understanding of the condition has changed and it is no longer seen as a disorder. No one's identity is a disorder; the diagnosis is based on the distress of body/mind incongruence. It is the distress caused by the dysphoria that is the disorder and is thus reflected in the DSM-5 criteria (Box 26.1).

Box 26.1 WPATH Depsychopathologization Statement (May 2010)

WPATH released a statement in May 2010 urging the depsychopathologization of gender nonconformity worldwide. This statement noted 'the expression of gender characteristics, including identities that are not stereotypically associated with one's assigned sex at birth, is a common and culturally diverse human phenomenon, which should not be judged as inherently pathological or negative'.

Box 26.2 Goal of the WPATH SOC (version 7)

The overall goal of the SOC is to provide clinical guidance for health professionals to assist transsexual, transgender and gender nonconforming people with safe and effective pathways to achieving lasting personal comfort with their gendered selves, in order to maximize their overall health, psychological well-being and self-fulfilment.

The current version of SOC (Version 7) acknowledges great variations in what health care provider will see. Many people with gender dysphoria will require some kind of medical intervention, but it will be tailored to their specific circumstance. For example, some will request hormones but no surgery; others might want chest surgery but no hormones and/or genital surgery, as examples (Box 26.2).

Transgender medical care

Unlike other areas of medicine where there is a clear aetiology and treatment algorithm, the aetiology of gender dysphoria is unknown. Medical care is based on symptomatology and the degree of relief of dysphoria with each intervention. Some people may transition socially whereas some may seek a medical transition with cross-sex hormone treatment and surgery (Box 26.3).

Medical interventions

Some individuals may require medical intervention to alleviate their gender dysphoria. These include cross-sex hormones and sex reassignment surgery also known as gender confirming surgery. As stated earlier, gender is no longer a binary concept and individuals will move along the gender spectrum to where they feel most comfortable.

Criteria for cross-sex hormones and gender affirming surgery

The WPATH SOC include guidelines for persons (adolescent and adult) wanting to have hormone (masculinizing and feminizing)

Box 26.3 Clinician Challenges

- There is no known aetiology of gender dysphoria.
- Epidemiology is fraught with research challenges and does not include estimates from the developing world.
- Most of the research literature is from North America and Western Europe.
- There are no physician findings nor lab tests to confirm the diagnosis. Successful diagnosis rests on the provider's clinical skills and the capacity of the patient for informed consent.
- The health care provider may not have encountered many trans people previously.
- Gender and transgender have multiple meanings contingent on culture and individual circumstance.
- Gender operates on a spectrum and trans clients can have multiple outcomes.

therapy and/or have surgery as part of their medical transition. An assessment and referral by a trained health care professional (HCP) in transgender health is required for these medical interventions.

Even though gender nonconformity is no longer seen as a mental disorder, as a result of stigma, pathologization, 'living with a secret', internalized transphobia and inadvertent faulty mirroring (not being socialized in authentic gender), many trans people have mental health concerns. Common ones include depression, anxiety, dissociation and substance abuse.

The HCP should have appropriate training and professional licensure in behavioural health and demonstrated competency in the assessment of gender dysphoria. This is particularly important when the HCP is functioning as part of a multidisciplinary specialty team that provides access to feminizing/masculinizing hormone therapy.

The goal of the assessment is to develop a care plan that is best suited to the needs of the individual. The clinician must be aware of other presentations that may mask as gender dysphoria where transition may not be in the best interest of the individual. These include psychosis and schizoaffective disorder with somatic delusions that disappear with psychotropic treatment, egodystonic homosexuality and compulsive cross-dressing.

Any adult wishing to start hormone therapy or breast/chest surgery must present with persistent, well-documented gender dysphoria; demonstrate the capacity to make a fully informed decision and to consent for treatment; and be the given age of majority in a given country. If significant medical or mental health concerns are present, documentation must support that these conditions are well managed. Although not an explicit criterion, it is recommended that male towards female (MtF) individuals undergo feminizing hormone therapy (minimum 12 months) before breast augmentation surgery. The purpose is to maximize breast growth in order to obtain better surgical (aesthetic) results. One letter from a qualified HCP is required for hormone therapy or breast/chest surgery.

In addition to the criteria set for hormone therapy and breast/surgery, 12 months of hormone therapy is recommended for removing fertility potential (gonadectomy). Continuous of living in a gender role that is congruent with the person's gender identity for 1 year is recommended for metoidioplasty or phalloplasty (neophallus) in female towards male (FtM) individuals and for vaginoplasty (neovagina) in MtF individuals. Two recommendation letters are required for genital surgery.

Feminizing/masculinizing hormone therapy

Some people with gender dysphoria will request hormone therapy as part of their medical transition and is considered medically necessary according to the WPATH SOC Version 7.

The following are the responsibilities of the prescribing physician:

1 Perform an initial evaluation that includes discussion of a patient's physical transition, goals, health history, physical examination, risk assessment and relevant laboratory tests.
2 Explain the effects and possible side effects including loss of reproductive potential.
3 Confirm that the patient has the capacity to consent for treatment.

4 Provide ongoing medical care include physical examinations and laboratory testing.
5 Provide necessary documentation to maximize patient safety (i.e. letters documenting hormone prescriptions etc.).

Feminizing and masculinizing hormone therapy

Typically feminizing hormone therapy is a combination of form of oestrogen and a testosterone blocker – either direct (cyproterone acetate) or indirect (spironolactone). Sometimes progesterone is added. Masculinizing therapy is initiated and maintained with testosterone. Gonadotrophin releasing hormone (GnRH) analogues are often used in youth for hormone blockade as a first step before cross-hormone therapy is prescribed.

Suggested dosing regimens and laboratory guidelines can be found in the WPATH SOC 7 and The Endocrine Society's *Guidelines for the Treatment of Transsexuals*.

Gender affirming surgery

Not all trans people will have surgery as part of their transition. Having said that, surgical modifications of the primary and/or secondary sex characteristics are medically necessary treatments to decrease gender dysphoria. Requirements set forth by the WPATH SOC for surgery have been described earlier. Options for feminizing surgery are found in Box 26.4 and masculinizing surgery in Box 26.5.

Box 26.4 **For the male-to-female (MtF) patient, surgical procedures may include the following:**

1 Breast/chest surgery: augmentation mammoplasty (implants/lipofilling);
2 Genital surgery: penectomy, orchiectomy, vaginoplasty, clitoroplasty, vulvoplasty;
3 Non-genital, non-breast surgical interventions: facial feminization surgery, liposuction, lipofilling, voice surgery, thyroid cartilage reduction, gluteal augmentation (implants/lipofilling), hair reconstruction, and various aesthetic procedures.

Box 26.5 **For the female-to-male (FtM) patient, surgical procedures may include the following:**

1 Breast/chest surgery: subcutaneous mastectomy, creation of a male chest;
2 Genital surgery: hysterectomy/ovariectomy, reconstruction of the fixed part of the urethra, which can be combined with a metoidioplasty or with a phalloplasty (employing a pedicled or free vascularized flap), vaginectomy, scrotoplasty, and implantation of erection and/or testicular prostheses;
3 Non-genital, non-breast surgical interventions: voice surgery (rare), liposuction, lipofilling, pectoral implants, and various aesthetic procedures.

In conclusion, people who present to a primary care provider will have medical needs like any one else and also needs that are trans specific such as requests for hormones. Trans people also may present with need for tests (such as a prostate examination for a trans woman, a cervical examination for a trans man) that are not regularly seen in their affirmed gender. It is important that the caregiver has a welcoming environment, non-judgemental stance and uses the pronoun and name consistent with the person's wishes.

Finally, living in a diverse world, HCPs must be sensitive to differences in cultural contexts and adapt the WPATH SOC Version 7 according to local realities.

Further reading

Hembree, W.C., Cohen-Kettenis, P., Delemarre-van de Waal, H.A. *et al.* (2009) Endocrine treatment of transsexual persons: an Endocrine Society clinical practice guideline. *Journal of Clinical Endocrinology and Metabolism*, **94** (**9**), 3132–3154.

Meyer-Bahlburg, H.F.L. (2010) From mental disorder to iatrogenic hypogonadism: dilemmas in conceptualizing gender identity variants as psychiatric conditions. *Archives of Sexual Behavior*, **39** (**2**), 461–476.

World Health Organization (2007) *International Classification of Diseases and Related Health Problems*, 10th Revision. World Health Organization, Geneva.

World Professional Association for Transgender Health (2012) *Standards of Care for the Health of Transsexual, Transgender, and Gender Nonconforming People*, 7th edn. World Professional Association for Transgender Health (WPATH), Minneapolis, MN. http://www.wpath.org/site_page.cfm?pk_association_webpage_menu=1351&pk_association_webpage=4655 (accessed 15/2/15).

WPATH Board of Directors (2010) Depsychopathologisation statement released May 26, 2010. Retrieved from http:// wpath.org/announcements_detail.cfm?pk_announcement.

Wylie, K., Barrett, J., Besser, M. *et al.* (2014) Good practice guidelines for the assessment and treatment of adults with gender dysphoria. *Sexual and Relationship Therapy*, **29** (**2**), 154–214.

CHAPTER 27

Psychosexual Therapy and Couples Therapy

Trudy Hannington

Leger Clinic, The College of Sexual and Relationship Therapists (COSRT), London, UK

OVERVIEW

The following chapter is an overview of psychosexual therapy and couples therapy giving an overview of sexual and relationship difficulties and possible therapeutic interventions.

Introduction

It is widely recognized that talking therapies can be extremely beneficial. In 2010, the UK government announced plans to make psychological therapies more available on the NHS.

Counselling/therapy allows a person to talk about their problems, concerns and feelings with a trained professional who listens with empathy. They can deal with negative thoughts and feelings in a non-judgemental way.

There are a number of different modalities used across counselling and therapy; the most common ones used in the field of sex and relationship therapy are described below.

Psychodynamic psychotherapy

This type of therapy is known as depth psychotherapy, it tends to focus on the unconscious and past experiences to establish why someone behaves the way they do now.

In this type of therapy, the focus would be on childhood relationships with parents and significant others in order to address difficult and challenging memories. Difficult childhood memories are often suppressed or denied and sit in the unconscious mind, the idea of psychodynamic psychotherapy is to address the negative and painful memories and feelings in order to let go and move on to form more constructive relationships with others.

Cognitive behavioural therapy

Cognitive behavioural therapy (CBT) is widely used, particularly within the NHS; it is based on helping an individual manage problems by changing the way a person thinks and feels.

CBT can be particularly useful in breaking a negative thought cycle. It focuses much more on the here and now (rather than the

past) and is broken down into small steps and achievable goals. CBT techniques help an individual challenge their thoughts and beliefs about themselves, other people and the world so that they no longer overgeneralize and magnify negative thoughts.

Cognitive restructuring

Cognitive restructuring is a core part of CBT and is used widely in sex therapy; common causes of sexual difficulties are often caused by incorrect or inadequate information resulting in unrealistic expectations.

This causes someone to have irrational beliefs about sex and often causes performance anxiety, by using cognitive restructuring people can learn to challenge their maladaptive thoughts and 'all or nothing' thinking.

Often a thought diary will be suggested to track negative and distorted thoughts and beliefs, the client is then encouraged to evaluate the evidence for/against those thoughts. The client is then encouraged to write a more balanced thought in order to challenge the distorted belief.

This can be particularly useful where anxiety is an issue in sex, for example painful sex, hypoactive sexual desire disorder (HSDD) and premature ejaculation used alongside a behavioural programme.

When a woman presents with a pain disorder or vaginismus, it often becomes a vicious circle (Figure 27.1) in which the perception of pain causes fear of pain which results in tension which in turn causes more pain.

The introduction of **BEHAVIOURAL TECHNIQUES** such as relaxation techniques and pelvic floor exercises (Kegel exercises) are particularly useful for sexual pain and vaginismus and there are specific techniques used for rapid ejaculation. These are described in Box 27.1.

PELVIC FLOOR EXERCISES (KEGEL EXERCISES) for men are an important factor, not only for maintaining strong muscle tone for good erections but also this can be particularly helpful for ejaculatory control. Learning to relax the pelvic floor and the buttocks can help delay ejaculation.

Relaxation and breathing exercises

Stress and anxiety have a huge impact on sexual functioning, learning specific relaxation techniques can be particularly useful.

ABC of Sexual Health, Third Edition. Edited by Kevan Wylie.
© 2015 John Wiley & Sons, Ltd. Published 2015 by John Wiley & Sons, Ltd.

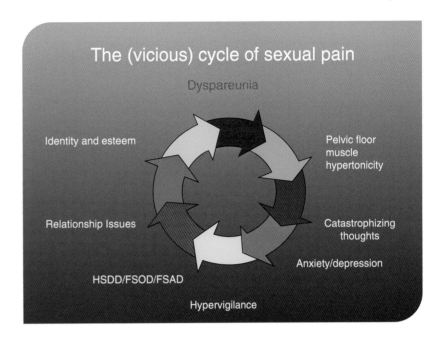

Figure 27.1 Vicious cycle of sexual pain

By learning to relax, a person will think more clearly and be able to focus much easier. Learning breathing techniques is the first step to the relaxation process;

Take a deep breath in and release slowly, repeat this a few times making sure the breathe is coming from the diaphragm not just the chest. Using relaxation CDs can really help and make the process easier, they often have background gentle music, waterfalls or waves gently rolling in the sea and some have guided fantasy which take you to pleasant places in order to relax a few levels deeper.

Even if you do not have much time a few deep breaths, dropping your shoulders and just slowing everything down a little can make a big difference. Taking yourself through each part of the body in turn, noticing any tension and gently letting it go. Exercise and fresh air will also help to ease anxiety and stress and in turn will give you more energy and help you to feel better about yourself.

The use of **SENSATE FOCUS**, a behavioural programme to remove the pressure of sex, was first introduced by Masters and Johnson in the 1970s, is particularly useful for couples who are finding sex difficult or just nonexistent.

Initially there is a 'ban' on sex and basic intimacy is introduced. There are many variations on this that are widely used in sex therapy today and are not always as prescriptive and regimented as it was in the 1970s in order to fit in with today's lifestyle. Nevertheless, it can be particularly useful if only used as a diagnostic tool to see where the couple are at in the relationship. The idea is to progress the basic intimacy from possibly agreeing and planning to spend some quality time together, holding hands and gentle kissing to much more intimate touching and 'date nights' guided by the therapist who will set homework and agree rules and boundaries for each stage of the intimacy process to keep the couples feeling safe and making steady progress. Gradually, the programme will become more intimate and more sexual from naked touching to progressing ad foreplay to full penetrative sexual activity.

Premature ejaculation if not being medically treated or alongside a medical intervention, a behavioural programme is introduced in sex therapy. **THE STOP/START TECHNIQUE** first introduced back in the 1950s consists of the masturbatory programme, where the man is encouraged to masturbate three to four times per week, using an arousal scale of 1–10 with a client can be particularly useful for him in order to become aware of the arousal process and the point of no return, and where he is on that arousal scale at any point during sexual activity. Initially, he would masturbate alone with a dry hand until he becomes aroused to mid-level about 5 and then stop for 10–15 s or until the arousal subsides slightly and then repeat the process again and on the third time to let go and enjoy ejaculation and orgasm learning to recognize the 'point of no return' in order to gain more control over the arousal process. This behavioural programme is then increased to introduce the partner. This process should also include encouraging a client to pay attention to the physical sensations in the penis and pelvic floor area rather than lasting longer, good relaxation of the pelvic floor is especially helpful in delaying ejaculation therefore a good awareness of any tension in the pelvic floor can be very beneficial.

THE SQUEEZE TECHNIQUE is where the penis is stimulated and either himself or his partner or squeezes the shaft of the penis between thumb and forefinger until the man loses his urge to ejaculate.

Mindfulness

Some groundbreaking work by 'Brotto' using mindfulness intervention for women with arousal disorder has shown excellent results and indeed mindfulness has been found to be an extremely effective treatment for many psychiatric and medical illness. There is more and more evidence to support the use of mindfulness techniques in psychosexual therapy (PST); the concept of mindfulness is about being 'present' in the moment. We often spend time thinking about what we have done or what we are going to do, rather than the moment we are in. Multitasking has become the norm! With sexual activity mindfulness can prevent someone 'spectatoring' and encourage him or her to participate by focusing on the sensations in their erogenous zones. By learning to tune out to negative or distracting thoughts and allow oneself to focus on the body's responses to sexual stimulation, it has been shown to demonstrate positive results.

PSYCHOSEXUAL THERAPY is a specific therapy to address a sexual dysfunction or a block between a couple preventing them from being sexual with one other.

Most psychosexual therapists will use an integrative approach usually including psychodynamic, behavioural and systemic as the basic principles. An important role for PST is to assess all of the potential risk factors as part of the initial assessment in history taking. Many individuals may have had a physiological factor that has caused the sexual dysfunction, however, by the time they seek help, which averages 2–3 years, it often has a psychological element too! Although there is much more media coverage about sex this does not necessarily mean that an individual or couple feel comfortable in talking about sexual matters.

It is vital that sexual difficulties are addressed as part of the couple relationship.

If a couple do not get on in the bedroom they often do not get on in the living room!!

Format of PST would include

- Assessment for suitability for PST
- History taking, to include family and sexual history and medical history
- Formulation
- Predisposing factors
- Precipitating factors
- Maintaining factors
- Establishing good rapport with the client
- Homework
- Consider Integrated Therapy (where appropriate)

Therapy should be individualized to meet the specific needs of the individual or couple. However, there are some basic principles and practices within the remit of PST, which differs from other therapy, and this is 'homework' for clients.

The initial session should include a complete history not only the sexual difficulty but of the relationship and each individual. The sexual relationship should be discussed in the context of the relationship as a whole. Any previous trauma/abuse must be addressed either in advance or alongside therapy. PST gives an opportunity for clients/patients to explore all aspects of their lives.

Systemic therapy

Systemic therapy was derived from family therapy and approaches problems in a practical way rather than in an analytical way. It allows an individual or a couple to identify their current patterns of behaviour in order to address the negative and stagnant patterns and introduce more positive interactions. This can be particularly useful for improving communication between couples.

EFFECTIVE COMMUNICATION is key to a successful relationship and a two-way process. This means being an active listener rather that a good talker!

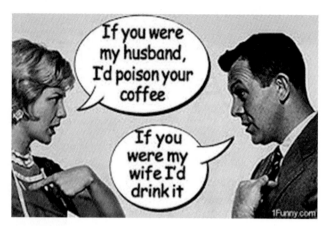

Figure 27.2 EFFECTIVE COMMUNICATION is key to a successful relationship. 1funny.com (public domain)

Most arguments for couples are caused through misunderstandings. The solution to stopping an argument before it starts is taking 'time out'.

As tempers flare (Figure 27.2), adrenalin increases and the body and mind then respond in 'fight or flight'. This results in either person being defensive, withdrawn, attacking or wanting to run. Although a simple technique, the use of 'I' at the beginning of each sentence can be an excellent way of stating clearly what the person is feeling or what the person would like, for example 'I feel close to you when … or I feel distant from you when … '

In many cases it can be extremmly helpful for an individual or couple to be given the opportunity to discuss their sexual difficulties and be offered reassurance, as to how common sexual difficulties can be.

The use of the PLISSIT model can be particularly useful in PST, it has four stages: Permission, Limited Information, Specific suggestions and Intensive therapy. This model was developed by Jack Annon and colleagues in 1974; the idea is that by going through each stage successfully in the above order the client goes on to a deeper level of treatment as they progress through each stage. However, it may not be necessary to go through each stage.

Permission, it is important to reassure a client at this stage that fantasy, sexual dreams, thoughts, feelings and behaviours are all normal (as long as they do not impact negatively on the partner). The focus on this stage is to reduce shame, anxiety and guilt. In some cases this may be all that is needed.

Limited Information, this is an opportunity for the therapist to explore myths and misconceptions about sex and give factual information, for example size of penis, orgasmic responses and effects of medication. Once again this may be all that is needed and the next stage may not be necessary.

Specific Suggestions, this is where 'homework' is introduced such as sensate focus or stop/start techniques. Helping a couple to improve the way they communicate and achieve goals.

Intensive Therapy, is needed where the sexual difficulty is caused by deeper relationship or underlying issues exist. There may be physical problems that need addressing with medical interventions or a psychiatric disorder such as depression, drug use and issues around sexuality will be a block to a client making progress and or being able to allow the client to complete homework tasks.

Social/interpersonal skills

Having good social/interpersonal skills really helps to build, maintain and enhance relationships with others. Having these skills enables a person to communicate and interact with others effectively. Practicing empathy can be very beneficial; this means being able to put oneself in another person's shoes to really consider how they may be feeling. Often conflict occurs from misunderstandings because people are not able to express themselves clearly or effectively; this causes frustration and leads to further conflict.

Body language is also important, giving another person good eye contact, smiling being calm and relaxed helps to keep someone's attention and helps them to feel at ease. Most people enjoy being around others who are happy, who communicate well, who show others that they genuinely care and are generally a positive person. Individuals with good social/interpersonal skills tend to be more successful both in their personal and professional life.

Myths

There are many common myths about sex! The following are some examples taken with kind permission of COSRT.

Here are a few commonly held beliefs about sex that you can safely ignore

- *The only true kind of sex involves someone putting their penis in someone else*
- *Having sex on your own is not really sex and it is bad to have sex on your own too much*
- *Sex should always involve an orgasm*
- *Sex should always start with lots of foreplay*
- *Foreplay is for kids*
- *Men need an erection in order to have sex*
- *Men should always initiate sex and should be in control of what happens*
- *Men are always ready for sex and always want it*
- *Women rarely want sex and need to be talked into it*
- *Men should be able to last all night*
- *Women should have sex with their partner otherwise they will lose them*
- *All kissing and touching should lead to sex*
- *You should never have sex on your own if you have a partner*
- *If you fantasize about someone else you are not happy with your partner*
- *If you have had sex with someone once you have to do it again*
- *If you have had one kind of sex it is not okay to say you do not want to do that any more*
- *Pornography accurately represents what great sex – and sexy bodies – really look like.*

Combined therapies

Whilst there are a number of validated psychotherapy treatments for sexual dysfunction more often than not a combination approach is what is necessary, integrated practice can be very beneficial for some sexual dysfunctions, integrating pharmacological products alongside sex therapy.

Although, an integrated approach for women is much more difficult given there are few limited pharmacological treatments available. The Eros Clitoral vice available for female arousal disorder can be beneficial. The use of conjugated equine oestrogen, approved and often used for the treatment of dyspareunia. There is also where and when appropriate the use of Hormone Replacement Therapy (HRT) and Topical testosterone for the treatment of HSDD.

MIST (Multi-intervention sex therapy)

Integrating approaches to sex therapy where more in depth treatment is needed, the MIST model is a good approach and offers a framework where medical and physical treatments, sex therapy techniques, cognitive-behavioural couple therapy and psychodynamic couple therapy are used in conjunction with one another and to compliment one another, giving an individual or couple a holistic approach to their presenting difficulties.

Use of bibliotherapy in sex therapy

Using bibliotherapy can be very useful in sex therapy, it helps a person resolve issues they have at the time or to relate to another person who has gone through the same thing. There are many self-help books and there is good evidence that these can play a positive role in the healing process.

A good example of this was the use of bibliotherapy as part of the treatment process for a group of women with vaginismus. The programme included sex education, relaxation, gradual exposure, cognitive therapy and sensate focus. Bibliotherapy was used throughout and good results were clearly evident from the study.

Hypnosis

For many years, hypnosis has been used with proven positive outcomes in sex therapy. Regression therapy can be used to uncover repressed memories; this enables a client to relive a difficult day or painful memory. The therapist would then use appropriate suggestions to help resolve them. Ego-strengthening in hypnotherapy provides hope and helps a client to recognize that positive change can occur. Hypnosis is often used as an adjunct to behavioural therapy; hypnosis is particularly helpful in aiding relaxation quickly and easily and helps facilitate positive visualization of good sexual activity. Visualization hypnotherapy is useful where anxiety and fear of failure is an issue regarding sexual activity. Positive imagery of successful sex where the therapist engages a client to not only visualize positive sexual activity but also enhance feelings and sensations in the body.

Additional resources used in addressing sexual problems

Many resources are available to use within sex therapy; however, it is important to take into account appropriateness and a good awareness of cultural and or religious beliefs so as not to offend a person or couple.

Use of erotica and bibliographies can be particularly useful. Erotic fiction, for example Fifty Shades of Grey and Black Lace are books to help with fantasy and arousal.

Vibrators have improved dramatically in recent years, they now come in various shapes, sizes, colours and materials; from very small bullet vibrators for clitoral stimulation to the traditional phallic shape vibrator for internal pleasure or the well known Rabbit that enhances both internal and external stimulation at the same time.

Lubricants – once again these have dramatically improved from the basic KY Jelly to oil-based, silicone and water-based; with pleasant smells and tastes.

Educational DVDs on lovemaking can be really useful for individuals and or couples for ideas, guidance and permission which some couples really welcome as there are a number of preconceived ideas about what people believe is ok and or acceptable sexually. "The lovers guide" collection and "Sex – A lifelong pleasures" are good examples.

Sex games, play things and Lingerie can be really useful for couples to gain confidence, get ideas and expand their repertoire in the bedroom. Dressing up for role-play together or just wearing sexy underwear can give a real boost to sexual confidence.

All of the above can now be bought easily either on the high street or through the Internet. Anne Summers and Pulse and Cocktails are now the norm in most towns and cities.

Where there is an underlying physical problem, there are medical devices for both men and women.

Dilators – to help retrain the vaginal muscle and response to penetration, these are used when a women has vaginismus or post vaginal surgery.

Eros device this is a small vacuum device helps stimulate blood flow to the clitoris in order to help arousal.

Vacuum devices and cock rings are a non-invasive treatment for men to gain an erection and help maintain it where an oral treatment is not possible or may have failed.

ones using electric currents (about £80 to £150). These devices can achieve quicker and better results.

To introduce basic techniques without using any devices, the following is a simple guide:

Initially it is important to locate the correct muscles, a good idea is to suggest a client/patient attempts to stop urinating mid-flow. (However, you would not recommend that they continue to do this as it can be harmful to the bladder.)

Step 1. Sit comfortably in a chair
Step 2. Squeeze the anus as though you are trying to stop a bowel movement and at the same time continue to tighten the vagina and urethra. It should feel as though you are attempting to hold everything 'up' inside.
Step 3. Hold the tension for 1 or 2 s and then relax so that you are tightening and relaxing quite quickly.
Step 4. Once you can do these exercises quite easily gradually hold the tension on each hold up to the count of 10.

Try to do 10 of these three times a day. Think breakfast, lunch and dinner to establish a good routine. It can also be beneficial to squeeze the pelvic floor muscles when coughing and sneezing to alleviate any further pressure.

Results are noticeable in just a few weeks.

Kegel exercises are also useful for women who experience painful sex and or vaginismus.

These women experience an involuntary spasm of the vagina – a protective guarding response. Introducing Kegel exercises can help to unlearn this response and learn to relax the pelvic floor muscles in order to enable penetration.

This will help the women to tolerate a vaginal examination, complete a smear test and enjoy penetrative sexual activity.

Vaginal dilators are often used for these type of conditions and can be helpful as part of this process. The most common used are Amielle and Femmax dilators. They come in different sizes, starting very small about the size of a finger and gradually increase in size to the size of an erect penis.

Self massage to the area or a vibrator can also be beneficial where painful sex is an issue or unprovoked vaginal pain is experienced.

Box 27.1 **Kegel exercises**

Kegel exercises were first discovered in 1948 by Dr Arnold Kegel. Kegels are exercises of the pelvic floor, the Pubococcygeus muscle that stretches from the pubic bone to the coccyx and supports the pelvic floor organs.

As people get older, after child birth, or pelvic floor surgery, pelvic floor muscles can become weaker, causing stress incontinence, prolapse, difficulties with sexual activity and weakened orgasm.

It is good practice to encourage clients/patients to do their pelvic floor exercises even if they do not experience any difficulties in order to prevent any future potential problems. However, where difficulties already exist it is not too late to introduce pelvic floor exercises, or refer to a specialist physiotherapist for specialist training, in some clinics pelvic floor trainers will be given on loan.

Pelvic floor trainers can also be bought in places like Boots or online, from very basic ones (about £30) to more sophisticated

Further reading

Brotto, L.A. *et al.*, (2008) A Mindfulness-Based group psychoeducational intervention targeting sexual arousal disorder in women. *Journal of Sexual Medicine*, **5**, 1646–59.

Brotto, L. (2013) Mindfulness & Sexuality (Special Issue) Sexual & Relationship Therapy, **28**, 1–152.

Bancroft, J. (2009) *Human Sexuality and its Problems (3rd Edition)*. Churchill Livingstone.

Barker, M. (2012) *Rewriting the rules*. Routledge.

Binik, Y.I. & Hall, K.S.K. (2014) *Principles & Practice of Sex Therapy 5th Edition*. Guilford Press.

De Carufel, F. & Trudel, G. (2006) Effects of a New Functional-Sexological treatment for premature ejaculation. *Journal of Sex and Marital Therapy*, **32**, 97–114.

EFS & ESSM Syllabus of Clinical Sexology (2013) *ESSM Education Committee*. Amsterdam: Medix Publishers.

ESSM Syllabus of Sexual Medicine (2012) *ESSM Educational Committee.* Amsterdam: Medix Publishers.

Hawton, K. (1985) *Sex Therapy: A Practical Guide.* Oxford Medical Publications.

Hudson-Allez, G. (1998) *Time Limited therapy.* Sage Publications.

Ford, V. (2010) *Overcoming sexual Problems.* London: Robinson.

Kleinplatz, P.J. (2012) *New directions in Sex Therapy.* New York: Routledge.

Luquet, W. (2006) *Short-Term Couples Therapy.* Routledge.

Recommended websites:
COSRT: cosrt.org.uk
NHS Choices: www.nhs.uk/Pages/HomePage.aspx
Relate: relate.org.uk
Porterbrook clinic: shsc.nhs.uk/porterbrook
UKCP: ukcp.org.uk

CHAPTER 28

Bibliotherapy and Internet-based Programmes for Sexual Problems

Jacques van Lankveld[1] and Fraukje E.F. Mevissen[2]

[1]Open University, Heerlen, The Netherlands
[2]Maastricht University, Maastricht, The Netherlands

OVERVIEW

- Self-help interventions range from simple informational solutions, via instructions for specific techniques to more complex interventions
- Bibliotherapy for sexual dysfunctions is moderately effective; treatment gains appear to diminish over time
- Therapist-assisted self-help is marginally more effective than unassisted self-help
- Video therapy is equally effective for female orgasmic problems as other self-help methods
- The efficacy of Internet-based therapy has received preliminary empirical support
- The Internet provides new opportunities for educational tools on sexual health
- The availability of online sexual health educational tools is large, but knowledge about their effectiveness still limited.

Introduction

Many women and men with sexual problems do not consult professionals for help. Some cannot, for various reasons, others do not want to. Although sexual problems are highly prevalent in the community, they are not easily revealed for reasons of embarrassment. Self-help interventions have certain advantages in this respect. They can accommodate the need for individuals with sexual problems to access professional services inconspicuously, securing privacy maintenance. The person's autonomy is better preserved than in face-to-face therapy, as there is less (emotional) dependence on a therapist. Moreover, because help is delivered in the home environment, there is no problem with the generalization of treatment gains to real-life situations. Finally, improvements in sexual functioning after self-help interventions can be better attributed to one's own competence, and thus boost one's self-esteem. Possible disadvantages of self-help approaches should also be recognized. Unsuccessful application of self-help strategies may diminish one's belief in the potential helpfulness of

professional sex therapy. Incorrect self-diagnosis may lead one to choose an unhelpful self-help strategy.

Not all sexual problems require professional involvement for their resolution, although chronic and complex sexual problems probably require more specialized and intensive professional help. Many sexual problems, especially in the early stage of development, can often be solved with minimal interventions. For instance, giving a woman, who experiences difficulty to have orgasms, permission to masturbate often solves the problem. Other problems require education on sexual anatomy and physiology, on normal ranges of sexual experiences, and so on. The next step in a stepped-care hierarchy involves giving specific suggestions, such as how to employ masturbation techniques, the use of lubricants, specific intercourse positions or the squeeze technique for premature ejaculation. Few problems are likely to require intensive professional help that includes sexual history taking, sensate focus training or cognitive restructuring.

The translation of professional-administered sex therapy to self-help and minimal-intervention forms of administration is probably more easily achieved than it is for many other mental health problems. Sex therapy has contained self-help elements ever since its emergence in the 1970s. The core ingredients of therapeutic change in sex therapy (the sensate focus exercises) have usually been performed in the privacy of the couples' homes. The only exception to this rule was the physician-sexologist or gynaecologist who assisted the female patient, when treating her vaginismus, with the vaginal insertion of dilators. We note that self-help or minimal interventions for other sexual disorders, such as paraphilic disorder or gender-identity disorder, are not found in the literature.

Types of self-help for sexual dysfunctions

Self-help interventions for sexual dysfunctions can be categorized by delivery format and can further be distinguished by amount of therapist contact. Bibliotherapy, video therapy and Internet-based sex therapy can be conducted with little or no therapist involvement. Telephone therapy, on its own or as an adjuvant to bibliotherapy or video therapy, and Internet therapy using digital exchange of messages require at least some involvement of a professional. These different venues for delivering self-help treatments are described in the following paragraphs; when possible, empirical evidence of their effectiveness is reported.

ABC of Sexual Health, Third Edition. Edited by Kevan Wylie.

Bibliotherapy

In bibliotherapy for sexual dysfunctions, written material is used to convey information on self-help techniques. The methods that are offered vary from recipe book-like protocols, that need to be followed in a stepwise fashion, to strategies that require the user to self-adapt a general problem-solving method to his or her personal conditions, and thus helps the user to become his or her own therapist. Mostly in these self-help books, techniques used in face-to-face therapy are translated into a self-help programme. They are based on methods developed by Masters and Johnson and from self-help approaches in cognitive therapy. Self-help manuals that are still commercially available in English were written by Barbach (2000), Heiman, LoPiccolo and LoPiccolo (1987) and Zeiss (1978). In the more recent manuals, cognitive restructuring receives more emphasis. Moderate to large effect sizes of treatment gains (ranging from 0.68 to 1.86 standard deviations) of bibliotherapy for various sexual dysfunction types were reported in meta-analyses. Unfortunately, post-treatment effects were found to erode over time. The included studies were largely limited to treatments for female and male orgasmic disorders. In a recent meta-analytic review (Van Lankveld, Hunot & Wylie, 2006), face-to-face sex counselling and minimal-contact self-help were found equally efficacious for men with premature ejaculation and women with orgasmic disorder.

Video therapy

Video therapy for sexual dysfunctions relies mainly on the principles of observational learning. The accompanying information usually covers the same topics as in bibliotherapy and face-to-face treatment, but the emphasis in video therapy is on observing a visual behavioural example first and then reproducing it in the participants' personal situation. Most video therapy formats follow the principles of sensate focus therapy. A small number of studies have been published of the effectiveness of video therapy. As an example, McMullen and Rosen (1979) compared videotape modelling with minimal therapist assistance to waiting-list control in pre-orgasmic women. Subjects in the video therapy watched a 20-min video tape. An actress portrayed a pre-orgasmic woman who learns to stimulate herself to orgasm and to transfer this newly acquired ability to sexual interaction with a partner. Sixty percent of the treated women became orgasmic, compared with none in the control group. Video therapies for other sexual dysfunctions have not been empirically tested.

Online sex therapy

Computer-assisted sex therapy can be delivered through the Internet, including online direct interaction of client and therapist, or it can be administered without human therapist involvement. Blended formats also exist, with a structured therapy programme encapsulated in a computer algorithm with a counsellor providing guidance. Both formats share many features of self-help: no face-to-face contact between client and therapist, strong privacy and autonomy features, no transportation time and costs. Interactive online sex therapy may be delivered synchronously, including direct (chat or audiovisual) contact or asynchronously through email contact. Many sex therapists have built easily traceable and accessible Web sites. Therapist-assisted, online sex therapy for male erectile disorder through e-mail with a cognitive-behavioural approach, including sensate focus exercises and cognitive restructuring, has been found efficacious, compared with waiting-list and active control groups. Average therapist time spent per treated participant ranges from about 1 to 4 h. A blended therapy with computerized treatment modules with adjuvant therapist email support for mixed female sexual dysfunctions yielded clinically significant improvements on all dimensions of sexual functioning.

Online educational tools for sexual health

The United Nations and the World Health Organization report that globally around 34 million people are living with HIV, while the total number of (curable) sexually transmitted infections (STIs) reached almost 500 million in 2008. In addition, 80 million women have unintended pregnancies of which more than half end in (regularly unsafe) abortions. Although these prevalence rates vary between countries and social groups (i.e. adolescents, men who have sex with men (MSM), intravenous drug users, sex workers and ethnic minorities), every sexually active person could be confronted with an STI or an unplanned pregnancy. In order to reduce those rates, health workers use different forms of sex education to motivate and help people to have no sex or safe sex (i.e. use condoms and contraception, and go for STI check ups).

One mode of delivering sexual health messages is via Internet. As access to the Internet is growing (USA rates reach 80%, Europe 63.2%), Internet-delivered sex education provides new opportunities to reach people in an anonymous way, with 24/7 accessibility, and mostly free of charge. Also, by using online health messages one may reach normally difficult-to-attain target groups. In addition, by using the Internet the message can be interactive and is easily tailored to the specific needs of a specific person and may thus partly replace expensive face-to-face sessions. These advantages are also in line with people's preferences to be in charge on *what* information they receive, *when*, and *how* they receive it. Finally, health messages that are tailored to the individual's needs also seem to be more effective.

When 'sex education' is entered in Google, one gets 726,000,000 hits in 0.34 s. Many of them will link you to sexual health information sites mostly delivered to you by municipal health centres, non-governmental organizations or (small) local health organizations from all over the world. The focus of these Web sites differs from sexual health and sexuality in general, to a specific focus on contraception, STI/HIV prevention or STI/HIV testing. The information provided on these Web sites ranges from basic information on STI's and pregnancy prevention (resembling brochures) to advanced Web sites with chat rooms or showing interactive videos with condom use instructions, tailored risk advice tools and sometimes even a message delivered in a virtual-reality world. However, even though Web sites may look very fancy or professional, it does not mean that the content or the form of the messages is theory- and evidence-based, nor does it mean that the messages are effective in helping people making healthy decisions or in changing their (unsafe) sexual behaviour. Moreover, several studies already showed that health (risk) messages can also have unintended opposite effects, even though its effectiveness seemed

Table 28.1 Brief selection of currently available sexual health education websites

URL	Target group	Content	Reference
www.langlevedeliefde.nl (press UK Flag for English version)	School going adolescents	Theory-based and proven effective school program on several sexual health issues. Partly available in English. Includes online and offline activities and materials such as a video (subtitled in English), a magazine, and a teacher manual.	Hofstetter, H., Peters, L.W.H., Meijer, S., VanKeulen, H.M., Schutte, L., VanEmpelen, P. (*in progress*). Evaluation of the effectiveness and implementation of the sexual health program long live love iv.
https://sph.uth.edu/iyg/	Middle school youth and HIV+ youth	Theory-based and evidence-based effective programs and applications on youth sexual health issues and HIV+ youth self-management skills. Includes online and offline activities.	Tortolero, S.R., *et al.* (2010). It's your game: Keep it real: Delaying sexual behavior with an effective middle school program. Journal of Adolescent Health, 46, 169–179
https://www.facebook.com /justusisis	Online youth	Peer and expert led effective Facebook intervention to promote condom use. Theory not mentioned.	Bull, S.S., Levine, D.K., Black, S.R., Schmiege, S.J., Santelli, J. (2012). Social Media-Delivered Sexual Health Intervention: A Cluster Randomized Controlled Trial. American Journal of Preventive Medicine, 43, 467–474
http://www.checkyourrisk .org.au/	Young people	Online tailored sexual risk advice and STI test recommendations. Theory not mentioned. No effects found.	Bilardi, J.E. *et al.*, (2009). The Experience of Providing Young People attending general practice with an online risk assessment tool to assess their own sexual risk. BMC Infectious Diseases, 9, doi:10.1186/1471-2334-9-29
http://www.hivbigdeal.org /HIVBIGDEAL2012/?event =page.index	18+ Men who have sex with men (MSM)	Online videos to increase serostatus disclosure and reduce unprotected anal intercourse among MSM. Theory-based and proven effectivity.	Hirshfield, S. *et al.*, (2012). An online randomized controlled trial evaluating HIV prevention digital media interventions for men who have sex with men. PLoS ONE, 7(10): e46252. doi:10.1371/journal.pone.0046252

logical (Mevissen, Meertens, Ruiter, Schaalma, 2010; Peters, Ruiter, Kok, 2013). So 'it cannot do any harm and it may do some good' can turn out very badly in this context.

Then which online educational tools for sexual health are effective? Unfortunately, this question can only partly be answered as just a minority of the world-wide available Web sites on sexual health has published evaluations in international peer-reviewed journals. However, we can also learn from looking at off-line programmes. Previous meta-analyses on the effectiveness of different health communication messages already showed that using so-called 'fear appeals', especially without including clear solutions, is not effective. Scaring people leads to high levels of fear and denial of the health message. In addition, it has been shown that there is very little evidence that abstinence programmes are effective. Programmes including multiple and interactive activities, including skills training, and using multiple sessions showed positive results (Kirby, 2002; Albarracín, Gillette, Earl, Glasman, Durantini, Ho, 2005). Finally, several meta-analyses on the effectiveness of online safer sex interventions showed that Web sites that are theory-based, Web sites including individualized messages and Web sites that did not only focus on knowledge (but, e.g. also include skills training) were more effective (among others: Noar, Pierce, Black, 2010). We have to note here, however, that a Web site's effectiveness also depends on whether the target group is reached and whether people spend sufficient time visiting it and taking in the messages. As 'workers in health', there is a shared responsibility to make people aware of the availability of these Web sites. For a brief selection of currently available Web sites see Table 28.1.

Further reading

Bartholomew, L.K., Parcel, G.S., Kok, G., Gottlieb, N.H. & Fernández, M.E. (2011) *Planning Health Promotion Programs: An Intervention Mapping Approach*. Jossey-Bass, San Francisco, CA.

Hucker, A. & McCabe, M.P. (2012) Manualized treatment programs for FSD: research challenges and recommendations. *Journal of Sexual Medicine*, **9**, 350–360.

Jones, L.M. & McCabe, M.P. (2011) The effectiveness of an internet-based psychological treatment program for female sexual dysfunction. *Journal of Sexual Medicine*, **8**, 2781–2792.

Mevissen, F.E.F., Ruiter, R.A.C., Meertens, R.M., Zimbile, F. & Schaalma, H.P. (2011) Justify your love: Testing an online STI-risk communication intervention designed to promote condom use and STI-testing. *Psychology & Health*, **26**, 205–221.

Noar, S.M., Clark, A., Cole, C. & Lustria, M.L.A. (2006) Review of interactive safer sex websites: practice and potential. *Health Communication*, **20**, 233–241.

Van Lankveld, J. (1998) Bibliotherapy in the treatment of sexual dysfunctions: a meta-analysis. *Journal of Consulting and Clinical Psychology*, **66**, 702–708.

Van Lankveld, J. (2009) Self-help therapies for sexual dysfunction. *Annual Review of Sex Research*, **46**, 143–155.

Van Lankveld, J., Wylie, K., van de Wetering, F. & Scholten, R. (under review). Bibliotherapy for sexual dysfunction. *Cochrane Database of Systematic Reviews*.

Van Lankveld, J., Leusink, P., van Diest, S. *et al.* (2009) Internet-based brief sex therapy for heterosexual men with sexual dysfunctions: a randomized controlled pilot trial. *Journal of Sexual Medicine*, **6**, 2224–2236.

CHAPTER 29

Sexual Pleasure

Sue Newsome

Sex Therapist & Tantra Teacher, London, UK

OVERVIEW
Key points include
- sexual pleasure as an approach to working with sexual issues
- influences and attitudes to sexual pleasure
- Sexual Confidence model for professionals.

Sexual pleasure

For students and professionals working in medicine and sexual health, the concept of sexual pleasure can be an extremely useful addition and enhancement to our professional toolkit. We have access to a wealth of accepted practices and protocols for identifying and treating sexual dysfunctions, but these give little or no consideration of whether the resulting sexual experience is actually enjoyable. It is increasingly recognized by professionals that sexual pleasure is an essential component of sexual health and wellbeing yet optimizing sexual function does not automatically guarantee good sex. If we focus solely on the patient's sexual dysfunction, we are not necessarily addressing their distress or difficulty. Consider women who have spent their adult life chasing an elusive orgasm and men who are feeling devastated about their failing erection, both will undoubtedly be euphoric when their sexual function improves but this elated state can quickly be replaced by dismay when they acknowledge that sex is still not enjoyable. When we ignore the question of sexual satisfaction, we run the risk of providing a short-term solution that does not fully address our patients' desire for satisfying sex lives.

Definition

Defining sexual pleasure presents a challenge, firstly it is a highly individual experience that has many determinants and influences and secondly it can significantly change due to a multitude of factors that include age and mood. Sexual pleasure can be experienced mentally as a fantasy or erotic thought, physically in response to sensual or sexual stimulation, emotionally with the feeling of togetherness with oneself or another, spiritually through deep connection

and may be a mix of all. If we accept the definition of sexual pleasure as 'positively valued feelings induced by sexual stimuli', it is no surprise that we do not have a universal scale to measure this diverse and multi-faceted human experience. By overlooking pleasure as one of the essential elements for satisfying sex, we fall into the trap of using indicators such as arousal, orgasm, ejaculation and intercourse to define a positive sexual experience. The belief that sexual function is synonymous with sexual pleasure may trigger performance anxiety which be an inhibiting factor on sexual function.

Influences and attitudes

Attitudes to sexual pleasure can vary enormously across cultures, religions, genders, abilities, sexual preferences and age groups. Our personal beliefs will determine whether we are comfortable with the idea of seeking enjoyment from sexual activity and the acceptable forms this may take. There is marked contrast between some Western religions that declare sex being exclusively for procreation and masturbation for sexual pleasure is sinful versus a spiritual practice such as Tantra (Figure 29.1), that celebrates all aspects of human sexuality and promotes the idea that human sexual pleasure can enjoyed as a spiritual experience.

Our culture and religion influence our beliefs, our developmental experiences create sexual imprints, modern media educates us about sexual norms and when we actually engage in sex with ourselves or another, we have to manage the interplay between our mind and body. An example of this is where the brain uses our beliefs about sexual norms to interpret sexual stimulation and influence our sexual response. For example, when a person who considers themselves to be heterosexual knows they are being touched intimately by someone of the same gender, their brain may interpret this as unacceptable but if they are blindfolded so they are unaware of the other person's gender, they may well experience pleasure.

Differences in attitude and approach to sexual pleasure can often underpin sexual problems. A patient reports inhibited orgasm and a discussion about sexual pleasure reveals that their lack of orgasm is actually because the stimulation they receive from their partner is ineffective and they lack the resources to ask for what they need, rather than there being any significant physical or psychological issue. Similarly, couples who complain about their non-existent sex lives may reveal that one of them is satisfied with regular, routine intercourse whereas their partner may desire more variety that

ABC of Sexual Health, Third Edition. Edited by Kevan Wylie.
© 2015 John Wiley & Sons, Ltd. Published 2015 by John Wiley & Sons, Ltd.

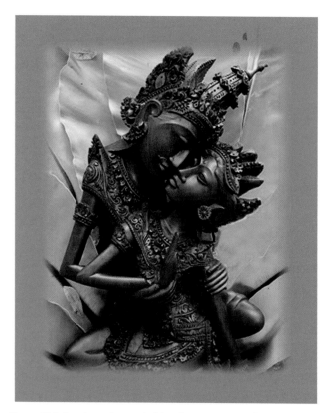

Figure 29.1 Tantric artefact symbolising the mystic union of male consciousness & female energy

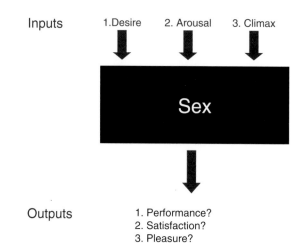

Figure 29.2 The 'black box' approach can be likened to giving our patients the ingredients to make a delicious cake & a photograph of the end result but leaving out the recipe & equipment that they need to make the cake (taken from APFELBAUM, Bernard (2012). On the need for a new sex therapy)

does not necessarily involve penetration and their avoidance of sex reflects their nervousness about discussing and negotiating their different sexual desires.

The eternal human quest to explore and create new possibilities for sexual pleasure is evidenced by the regular emergence of new sexual practices, fetishes and behaviours as well as recycling of long-forgotten ones. For example, the Victorian interest in figging (the insertion of root ginger into the anal or vaginal opening) is currently enjoyed as one of the more unusual practices within BDSM (Bondage, Discipline, Domination, Submission, Sado-Masochism). The myriad of options to attain sexual pleasure highlights the need for sexual health professionals to understand current trends in sexual behaviour. We must be aware of our own attitudes towards sex in order to minimize the risk of making assumptions about how our patients may derive their sexual pleasure and not let our personal judgements to negative impact on our work. One person's sexual pleasure can seem irritating, boring or abhorrent to someone else.

An increasing risk for professionals is that we are seduced by the advances in sexual medicine into adopting a 'black box' approach (Figure 29.2) when working with sexual issues. This occurs when we assume that the necessary inputs for satisfying sexual activity are desire, arousal and climax and our methodology consists of making a prompt diagnosis of a sexual dysfunction, offering a treatment plan that is solely focused on achieving sexual function and when this happens, we tick the box for a positive outcome. Using this approach, we are leaving it to the patients to navigate the 'black box' of solo or partnered sex and furthermore we are assuming that

because they have sexual function, they will automatically achieve a satisfactory outcome from any sexual interaction. Undoubtedly a patient's distress about an absent or failing aspect of their sexual response is replaced by immense relief when function is achieved or restored but this can quickly become despair if sex continues to be disappointing or unsatisfactory for them.

The sexual act between adults is described as a complex social interaction governed by social rules that, above all, require both honest communication and willingness to be vulnerable for true intimacy and pleasure to occur. When patients do not have experience of the language, skills and behaviours that support mutual pleasure, they often describe their sexual interactions as events to survive, endure or 'put up with'. The idea of 'speaking the unspeakable' and communicating the truth of what is happening for them is totally contrary to the popular belief that, if we feel desire and can achieve arousal, we are guaranteed a fantastic experience. We have the opportunity to offer guidance, education and skills that can equip patients to explore and enjoy the mystery of the 'black box' of their sexual encounters.

A measure for pleasure

The provision of robust, comprehensive sex education goes a long way to supporting healthy sexual attitudes and sexual enjoyment. Current UK sex education is narrowly focused on prevention of sexually transmitted infections (STIs) and unwanted pregnancy and, although it is usually the strong drive for pleasure that causes people to explore sex with themselves or others, current education lacks any constructive teachings about the reality and potential pleasure of the human sexual experience. Consequently, we are educated by the media and pornography where the pervading messages include men have large genitals, women have pert breasts, partnered sex always involves penetration and simultaneous orgasm and solo sex must include a climax for it to be worthwhile. Interestingly, much of the sexual imagery available portrays sexual activity between two or more people which implies that partnered sex is the only way to

The pleasure perspective

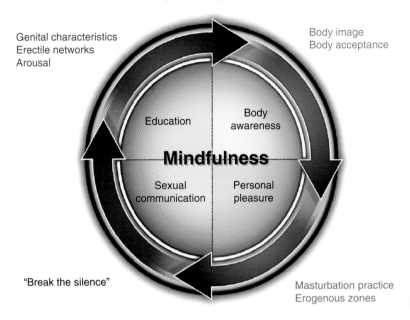

Genital characteristics
Erectile networks
Arousal

Body image
Body acceptance

"Break the silence"

Masturbation practice
Erogenous zones

Figure 29.3 Sexual Confidence Model

achieve pleasure and that another person is required to validate our sexuality and sexual prowess. This commentary on masturbation; a regular and accepted practice for most many, perpetuates the stigmatization of an activity which has significant potential for pleasure.

Sexual stereotypes and goal-oriented sex are easily adopted as ideals and this naturally gives rise to comparisons which can have an extremely negative impact on body image and cause patients to feel inadequate, ashamed and dissatisfied with themselves and their sex life. Also our cultural reluctance to talk honestly and openly about sex simply maintains the myths believed by many; that is everyone else is having more sex than me, everyone else is better at sex than me and they are all enjoying it more than I am!

Sexual confidence

Without doubt, one of the most powerful interventions we can make is to help our patients define sexual pleasure for themselves. There are a number of possibilities for professionals to incorporate sexual pleasure into their work with sexual concerns:

- The initial assessment process can include specific questions relating to sexual pleasure and medical and psychological interventions can be enhanced to ensure that the formulation and overall outcome is focused on pleasure. Patients can be asked to rate their current level of sexual pleasure and describe the level and quality of pleasure they desire.
- Once sexual function is achieved or restored, sexual pleasure can be included as an extra step in the treatment process.
- In certain cases, sexual pleasure can be used as an alternative approach to completely take the emphasis away from performance so that patients are more able to accept and enjoy

their level of sexual function even when it does match their expectations or ideals.

Including questions about sexual pleasure as part of the initial assessment can quickly open up frank discussions about the reality of human sexual activity in that it can be clumsy, funny, exhilarating, pleasurable, disappointing, surprising and so much more. The Sexual Confidence model (Figure 29.3) provides a useful framework for professionals to design a simple programme specific to each patient. It can increase sexual confidence and encourage the patient to take responsibility for their sexual pleasure rather than being obsessed with performance. Using this model, a presenting problem can be easily transformed into a personal pleasure plan.

The four elements of the Sexual Confidence model are:

1 Education
  This includes the provision of realistic facts and statistics on adult body shape, genital characteristics, erectile networks in male and female genital anatomy and sexual arousal cycles. Photographs and illustrations are used to normalize differences in human genital anatomy.
2 Body awareness
  A series of exercises, including relaxation, to address ambivalent and negative body image and develop increased body awareness and acceptance. This aspect is particularly important for patients with chronic illness or physical disability.
3 Personal pleasure
  This aspect of the model involves the development of a pleasure-based (rather than goal-focused) masturbation practice. The objective is to re-frame masturbation, significantly expand the possibilities for self-pleasure and explore sexual arousal. Enhanced mindfulness as a discipline can encourage

full consciousness and presence. Greater understanding of personal pleasure can then be applied to inform and enhance partnered sex. A further step is to explore different sexual desires and expressions, for example, fantasies, fetishes and unfulfilled sexual yearnings.

4 Sexual communication

This includes specific communication techniques to break the silence that so often occurs around sexual activity and to allow for heartfelt articulation and communication of sexual needs and desires, with the result of increased intimacy.

Introducing sexual pleasure provides a different dimension to working with sexual issues and opens up possibilities for achieving a positive outcome in a relatively short period of time. One of the most significant contributions we can make in the field of sexual health and sexual medicine is to encourage our patients to let go of unrealistic performance goals and unhelpful comparisons, inspire them to define and celebrate their sexual pleasure and help them to acknowledge that their sexual pleasure is personal, dynamic and diverse.

Further reading

Apfelbaum, B. (2012) On the need for a new direction in sex therapy. In: Kleinplatz, P.J. (ed), *New Directions in Sex Therapy Innovations and Alternatives*. Routledge, New York, pp. 5–20.

Carrellas, B. (2007) *Urban Tantra: Sacred Sex for the Twenty-First Century*. Celestial Arts, Berkeley.

Okan, M. (2012). *Feminine Beauty: A Celebration*. Spirit Fire Productions, Phoenix.

Okan, M. (2012). *Masculine Power: A Tribute*. Spirit Fire Productions, Phoenix.

Perel, E. (2007) *Mating in Captivity: Sex, Lies and Domestic Bliss*. Hodder and Stoughton, London.

Schnarch, D. (2009) *Intimacy and Desire: Awaken the Passion in Your Relationship*. Beaufort Books, New York.

Sommers, F.G. (2013) Mindfulness in love and love making: a way of life. *Sexual and Relationship Therapy*, **28**, 84–91.

Winston, S. (2010). *Women's Anatomy of Arousal*. Mango Garden Press, New York.

Index

Note: Page numbers in *italics* refer to Figures; those in **bold** to Tables

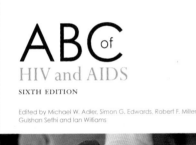

ABC of Breast Diseases

4TH EDITION

J. Michael Dixon
Western General Hospital, Edinburgh, UK

Breast diseases are common and often encountered by health professionals in primary care. While the incidence of breast cancer is increasing, earlier detection and improved treatments are helping to reduce breast cancer mortality. The *ABC of Breast Diseases, 4th Edition*:

- Provides comprehensive guidance to the assessment of symptoms, how to manage common breast conditions and guidelines on referral
- Covers congenital problems, breast infection and mastalgia, before addressing the epidemiology, prevention, screening and diagnosis of breast cancer and outlines the treatment and management options for breast cancer within different groups
- Includes new chapters on the genetics, prevention, management of high risk women and the psychological aspects of breast diseases
- Is ideal for GPs, family physicians, practice nurses and breast care nurses as well as for surgeons and oncologists both in training and recently qualified as well as medical students

AUGUST 2012 | 9781444337969 | 168 PAGES | £27.99/US$46.95/€35.90/AU$52.95

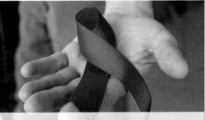

ABC of HIV and AIDS

6TH EDITION

Michael W. Adler, Simon G. Edwards, Robert F. Miller, Gulshan Sethi & Ian Williams
University College London Medical School; Mortimer Market Centre, London; University College London; St Thomas' Hospital, London Medical School; University College London Medical School

Since the previous edition, big advances have been made in treatment, knowledge of the disease and epidemiology. The problem of AIDS in developing countries has become a major political and humanitarian issue.

- Edited by the Director of the Department for Sexually Transmitted Diseases, *ABC of HIV and AIDS, 6th Edition* is an authoritative guide to the epidemiology, incidence, and most up to date management of HIV and AIDS
- Reflects the constantly changing knowledge of the disease and its manifestations, new developments in drug and non-drug management, sociological and political issues
- Includes 6 new chapters on conditions associated with AIDS and further concentration on the community effects of the disease, and the situation of women with AIDS
- Ideal for all levels of health care workers caring for HIV and AIDS patients

JUNE 2012 | 9781405157001 | 144 PAGES | £24.99/US$49.95/€32.90/AU$47.95

ABC of Pain

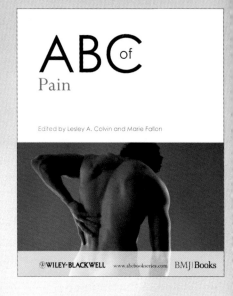

Lesley A. Colvin & Marie Fallon
Western General Hospital, Edinburgh; University of Edinburgh

Pain is a common presentation and this brand new title focuses on the pain management issues most often encountered in primary care. *ABC of Pain*:

- Covers all the chronic pain presentations in primary care right through to tertiary and palliative care and includes guidance on pain management in special groups such as pregnancy, children, the elderly and the terminally ill
- Includes new findings on the effectiveness of interventions and the progression to acute pain and appropriate pharmacological management
- Features pain assessment, epidemiology and the evidence base in a truly comprehensive reference
- Provides a global perspective with an international list of expert contributors

JUNE 2012 | 9781405176217 | 128 PAGES | £24.99/US$44.95/€32.90/AU$47.95

ABC of Urology

3RD EDITION

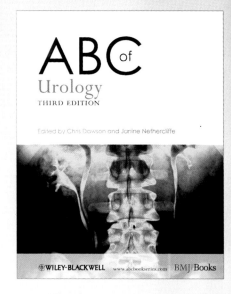

Chris Dawson & Janine Nethercliffe
Fitzwilliam Hospital, Peterborough; Edith Cavell Hospital, Peterborough

Urological conditions are common, accounting for up to one third of all surgical admissions to hospital. Outside of hospital care urological problems are a common reason for patients needing to see their GP.

- *ABC of Urology, 3rd Edition* provides a comprehensive overview of urology
- Focuses on the diagnosis and management of the most common urological conditions
- Features 4 additional chapters: improved coverage of renal and testis cancer in separate chapters and new chapters on management of haematuria, laparoscopy, trauma and new urological advances
- Ideal for GPs and trainee GPs, and is useful for junior doctors undergoing surgical training, while medical students and nurses undertaking a urological placement as part of their training programme will find this edition indispensable

MARCH 2012 | 9780470657171 | 88 PAGES | £23.99/US$37.95/€30.90/AU$47.95

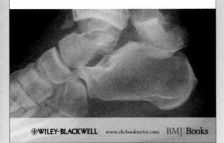

ABC of Emergency Radiology

3RD EDITION

Otto Chan
London Independent Hospital

The *ABC of Emergency Radiology, 3rd Edition* an invaluable resource for accident and emergency staff, trainee radiologists, medical students, nurses, radiographers and all medical personnel involved in the immediate care of trauma patients.

- Follows a systematic approach to assessing radiographs
- Each chapter covers a different part of the body, leading through the anatomy for ease of use
- Includes clear explanations and instructions on the appearances of radiological abnormalities with comparison to normal radiographs throughout
- Incorporates over 400 radiographs

JANUARY 2013 | 9780470670934 | 144 PAGES | £29.99/US$48.95/€38.90/AU$57.95

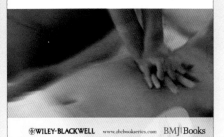

ABC of Resuscitation

6TH EDITION

Jasmeet Soar, Gavin D. Perkins & Jerry Nolan
Southmead Hospital, Bristol; University of Warwick, Coventry; Royal United Hospital, Bath

A practical guide to the latest resuscitation advice for the non-specialist *ABC of Resuscitation, 6th Edition*:

- Covers the core knowledge on the management of patients with cardiopulmonary arrest
- Includes the 2010 European Resuscitation Council Guidelines for Resuscitation
- Edited by specialists responsible for producing the European and UK 2010 resuscitation guidelines

DECEMBER 2012 | 9780470672594| 144 PAGES | £28.99/US$47.95/€37.90/AU$54.95

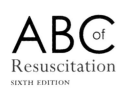

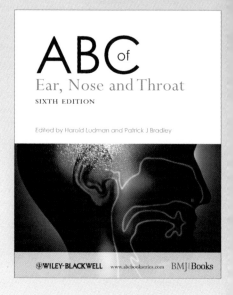
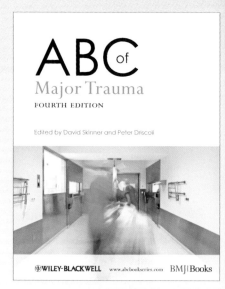

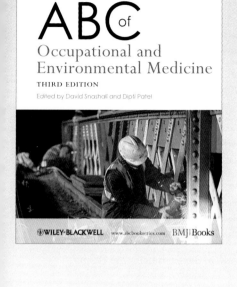

ABC of Occupational and Environmental Medicine

3RD EDITION

David Snashall & Dipti Patel

Guy's & St. Thomas' Hospital, London; Medical Advisory Service for Travellers Abroad (MASTA)

Since the publication of last edition, there have been huge changes in the world of occupational health. It has become firmly a part of international public health, and in Britain there is now a National Director for Work and Health. This fully updated new edition embraces these changes and:

- Provides comprehensive guidance on current occupational and environmental health practice and legislation
- Concentrates on the newer kinds of occupational disease, for example 'RSI', pesticide poisoning and electromagnetic radiation, where exposure and effects are difficult to understand
- Places an emphasis on work, health and well-being, and the public health benefits of work, the value of work, disabled people at work, the aging workforce, and vocational rehabilitation
- Includes chapters on the health effects of climate change and of occupational health and safety in relation to migration and terrorism

NOVEMBER 2012 | 9781444338171 | 168 PAGES | £27.99/US$44.95/€38.90/AU$52.95

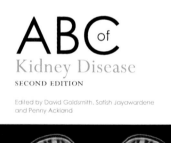
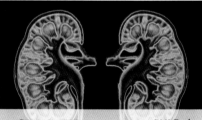

ABC of Kidney Disease

2ND EDITION

David Goldsmith, Satish Jayawardene & Penny Ackland

Guy's & St. Thomas' Hospital, London; King's College Hospital, London; Melbourne Grove Medical Practice, London

Nephrology is sometimes considered a complicated and specialized topic and the illustrative ABC format will help GPs quickly and easily assimilate the information needed. *ABC of Kidney Disease, 2nd Edition*:

- Is a practical guide to the most common renal diseases to enable non-renal health care workers to screen, identify, treat and refer renal patients appropriately and to provide the best possible care
- Covers organizational aspects of renal disease management, dialysis and transplantation
- Provides an explanatory glossary of renal terms, guidance on anaemia management and information on drug prescribing and interactions
- Has been fully revised in accordance with new guidelines

OCTOBER 2012 | 9780470672044 | 112 PAGES | £27.99/US$44.95/€35.90/AU$52.95